Medical Quotes
A Thematic Dictionary

EDITED BY

JOHN DAINTITH
and
AMANDA ISAACS

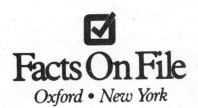

Facts On File
Oxford • New York

Medical Quotes
A Thematic Dictionary

Facts on File, Ltd.
Collins Street
Oxford OX4 1XJ
United Kingdom

or

Facts on File, Inc.
460 Park Avenue South
New York NY 10016
USA

Medical Quotes

1. Medicine
I. Daintith, John   II. Isaacs, Amanda
610

ISBN 0-8160-2094-9

Library of Congress CIP data available on request

Compiled and typeset by Market House Books Ltd., Aylesbury
Text design by CGS Studios, Cheltenham
Jacket design by CGS Studios, Cheltenham
Printed in Great Britain by Billing & Sons Ltd, Worcester

10 9 8 7 6 5 4 3 2 1

This book is printed on acid-free paper.

INTRODUCTION

The dictionary of quotations is a compilation of writings, sayings, and remarks about medicine and related subjects.

We have arranged the quotations under themes. Within each entry the quotations are in alphabetical order of the author's surname. Cross references are given to related topics, but in a few cases, in which a quote is particularly appropriate to two different topics, we have duplicated it.

In choosing the theme headings we have concentrated on topics of general interest, rather than on specialist subjects. There may well be interesting, perceptive, or witty remarks about Wernicke's encephalopathy or Henle's loop – but you will not find them here. The topics are general ones – medicine, disease, drugs, birth, old age, death, doctors, nurses, and, of course, patients.

Each quotation is followed by the author's name, dates, and a short biography, with a source reference for the quotation. In some cases we have been unable to find some or all of this information. However, we have still included the quote, taking the view that the reader would prefer an incomplete entry to nothing at all. We would be grateful to any readers who can supply any missing information.

We have included two indexes in the book. The first is a keyword – key phrase index, which will help the user to locate a half-remembered quotation or to find the source of a known one. The reference in the index is to the theme and to the number of the quote within that theme. The second index is an index of authors, similarly arranged.

We hope that these indexes will make this a useful reference book. But, above all, we hope that the book itself will provide interesting and sometimes amusing reading for doctors and patients alike.

The Editors

A

ABORTION

1   Some women behave like harlots; when they feel the life of a child in their
    wombs, they induce herbs or other means to cause miscarriage, only to per-
    petuate their amusement and unchastity. Therefore I shall deprive them from
    everlasting life and send them to everlasting death.
    Bridget of Sweden (1303–73) Swedish nun and visionary.
    Revelations, Vol. VII

2   Abortion leads to an appalling trivialization of the act of procreation.
    Donald Coggan, Archbishop of York (1909–   ) British churchman.
    Speech to the Shaftesbury Society, 2 Oct 1973

3   It serves me right for putting all my eggs in one bastard.
    Dorothy Parker (1893–1967) US writer and wit.
    You Might As Well Live, II, Ch. 3 (J. Keats)
    On going into hospital for an abortion

4   The greatest destroyer of peace is abortion because if a mother can kill her
    own child what is left for me to kill you and you to kill me? There is noth-
    ing between.
    Mother Teresa (1910–   ) Yugoslavian missionary in Calcutta.
    Nobel Peace Prize Lecture

5   To hinder a birth is merely speedier man-killing; nor does it matter whether
    you take away a life that is born, or destroy one that is coming to the birth.
    That is a man which is going to be one; you have the fruit already in its
    seed.
    Tertullian (c. 160–c. 225) Carthaginian father of the church.
    Apologeticus, IX

6   If a man come near unto a damsel, . . . and she conceives by him, and she
    says, 'I have conceived by thee;' and he replies, 'Go then to the old woman
    and apply to her that she may procure thee miscarriage;'
    And the damsel goes to the old woman and applies to her that she may pro-
    cure her miscarriage; and the old woman brings her some Banga or Shaêta, or
    Ghnâna or Fraspâta, or some other of the drugs that produce miscarriage and
    the man says, 'Cause thy fruit to perish!' and she causes her fruit to perish;
    the sin is on the head of all three, the man, the damsel, and the old
    woman.
    The Zend-Avesta (c. 550 BC)
    The Vendidad, XV:2

ABSTINENCE
See also **DRINKING, SEX, SMOKING.**

1 If you resolve to give up smoking, drinking and loving, you don't actually live longer; it just seems longer.
Anonymous

2 He neither drank, smoked, nor rode a bicycle. Living frugally, saving his money, he died early, surrounded by greedy relatives. It was a great lesson to me.
John Barrymore (1882–1942) US actor.
The Stage, Jan 1941 (J. P. McEvoy)

3 I must point out that my rule of life prescribes as an absolutely sacred rite smoking cigars and also the drinking of alcohol before, after, and if need be during all meals and in the intervals between them.
Winston Churchill (1874–1965) British statesman.
The Second World War
Said during a lunch with the Arab leader Ibn Saud, when he heard that the king's religion forbade smoking and alcohol

4 Teetotallers lack the sympathy and generosity of men that drink.
W. H. Davies (1871–1940) British poet.
Shorter Lyrics of the 20th Century, Introduction

5 It was a brilliant affair; water flowed like champagne.
William M. Evarts (1818–1901) US lawyer and statesman.
Describing a dinner given by US President Rutherford B. Hayes (1877–81), an advocate of temperance
Attrib.

6 Mr. Mercaptan went on to preach a brilliant sermon on that melancholy sexual perversion known as continence.
Aldous Huxley (1894–1964) British writer.
Antic Hay, Ch. 18

7 The few bad poems which occasionally are created during abstinence are of no great interest.
Wilhelm Reich (1897–1957) Austrian-born US psychiatrist.
The Sexual Revolution

8 Temperance is the love of health, or the inability to overindulge.
Duc François de La Rochefoucauld (1613–80) French writer.
Maxims, No. 583

9 The people who are regarded as moral luminaries are those who forego ordinary pleasures themselves and find compensation in interfering with the pleasures of others.
Bertrand Russell (1872–1970) British philosopher.
Sceptical Essays

10 Lastly (and this is, perhaps, the golden rule), no woman should marry a tee-
    totaller, or a man who does not smoke.
    Robert Louis Stevenson (1850–94) Scottish writer.
    Virginibus Puerisque

11 Though in silence, with blighted affection, I pine,
    Yet the lips that touch liquor must never touch mine!
    G. W. Young (19th century) British writer.
    The Lips That Touch Liquor

ACCIDENTS

1 ACCIDENT n. An inevitable occurrence due to the action of immutable
   natural laws.
   Ambrose Bierce (1842–c. 1914) US writer and journalist.
   The Devil's Dictionary

2 The Act of God designation on all insurance policies; which means, roughly,
   that you cannot be insured for the accidents that are most likely to happen
   to you.
   Alan Coren (1938–) British humorist and writer.
   The Lady from Stalingrad Mansions, 'A Short History of Insurance'

3 Knocked down a doctor? With an ambulance? How could she? It's a contra-
   diction in terms.
   N. F. Simpson (1919–) British dramatist.
   One-Way Pendulum, I

4 The chapter of accidents is the longest chapter in the book.
   John Wilkes (1725–97) English politician.
   Attrib. in *The Doctor* (Southey), Vol. IV

ADDICTION
See also **DRINKING, NARCOTICS, SMOKING.**

1 Every form of addiction is bad, no matter whether the narcotic be alcohol or
   morphine or idealism.
   C. G. Jung (1875–1961) Swiss psychoanalyst.
   Memories, Dreams, Reflections, Ch. 12

ADOLESCENCE
See **YOUTH.**

AGE
See also **LONGEVITY, MIDDLE AGE, OLD AGE, YOUTH.**

1 Man arrives as a novice at each age of his life.
Nicolas Chamfort (1741–94) French writer and wit.
Caractères et anecdotes, 576

2 A man is as old as he's feeling,
A woman as old as she looks.
Mortimer Collins (1827–76) British writer.
The Unknown Quantity

3 The years that a woman subtracts from her age are not lost. They are added
to the ages of other women.
Diane de Poitiers (1499–1566) French courtesan.
Attrib.

4 Youth is a blunder; manhood a struggle; old age a regret.
Benjamin Disraeli, Lord Beaconsfield (1804–81) British statesman.
Coningsby, Bk. III, Ch. 1

5 The years between fifty and seventy are the hardest. You are always being
asked to do things, and you are not yet decrepit enough to turn them down.
T. S. Eliot (1888–1965) US-born British poet and dramatist.
Time, 23 Oct 1950

6 At sixteen I was stupid, confused, insecure and indecisive. At twenty-five I
was wise, self-confident, prepossessing and assertive. At forty-five I am stupid,
confused, insecure and indecisive. Who would have supposed that maturity is
only a short break in adolescence?
Jules Feiffer (1929–) US writer, cartoonist, and humorist.
The Observer, 3 Feb 1974

7 She may very well pass for forty-three
In the dusk, with a light behind her!
W. S. Gilbert (1836–1911) British dramatist.
Trial by Jury

8 We do not necessarily improve with age: for better or worse we become more
like ourselves.
Peter Hall (1930–) British theatre director.
The Observer, 'Sayings of the Week', 24 Jan 1988

9 The four stages of man are infancy, childhood, adolescence and obsolescence.
Art Linkletter (1912–) Canadian-born US radio and television personality.
A Child's Garden of Misinformation, 8

10 I am just turning forty and taking my time about it.
Harold Lloyd (1893–1971) US silent-film comedian.
Reply when, aged 77, he was asked his age
The Times, 23 Sept 1970

11 Do you think my mind is maturing late,

Or simply rotted early?
Ogden Nash (1902–71) US poet.
Lines on Facing Forty

12   A man need not look in your mouth to know how old you are.
     Proverb

13   Men come of age at sixty, women at fifteen.
     James Stephens (1882–1950) Irish novelist.
     The Observer, 'Sayings of the Week', 1 Oct 1944

14   A man is as old as his arteries.
     Thomas Sydenham (1624–89)
     Bulletin of the New York Academy of Medicine, 4:993, 1928 (F. H. Garrison)

15   Life begins at forty.
     Sophie Tucker (Sophia Abuza; 1884–1966) Russian-born US singer and vaude-
     ville star.
     Attrib.

16   From birth to age eighteen, a girl needs good parents. From eighteen to
     thirty-five, she needs good looks. From thirty-five to fifty-five, she needs a
     good personality. From fifty-five on, she needs good cash.
     Sophie Tucker
     Attrib.

AIDS

1   Everywhere I go I see increasing evidence of people swirling about in a
    human cesspit of their own making.
    James Anderton (1932–) British Chief Constable of Greater Manchester.
    Referring to AIDS

2   It could be said that the Aids pandemic is a classic own-goal scored by the
    human race against itself.
    Princess Anne (1950–) The Princess Royal, only daughter of Elizabeth II.
    Remark, Jan 1988

3   My message to the businessmen of this country when they go abroad on busi-
    ness is that there is one thing above all they can take with them to stop
    them catching AIDS, and that is the wife.
    Edwina Currie (1946–) British politician.
    The Observer, 15 Feb 1987

4   We're all going to go crazy, living this epidemic every minute, while the rest
    of the world goes on out there, all around us, as if nothing is happening, go-
    ing on with their own lives and not knowing what it's like, what we're going

through. We're living through war, but where they're living it's peacetime, and we're all in the same country.
Larry Kramer (1935–) US dramatist and novelist.
The Normal Heart

ALCOHOL
See **DRINKING.**

ALLERGIES

1 We've made great medical progress in the last generation. What used to be merely an itch is now an allergy.
Anonymous

ANAESTHESIA

1 And the Lord God caused a deep sleep to fall upon Adam, and he slept: and he took one of his ribs, and closed up the flesh instead thereof.
Bible: Genesis
2:21

2 Three natural anaesthetics . . . sleep, fainting, death.
Oliver Wendell Holmes (1809–94) US writer and physician.
Medical Essays, 'The Medical Profession in Massachusetts'

3 Dr. Simpson's first patient, a doctor's wife in 1847, had been so carried away with enthusiasm that she christened her child, a girl, 'Anaesthesia'.
Elizabeth Longford (1906–) British writer.
Queen Victoria, Ch. 17

4 Mr. Anaesthetist, if the patient can keep awake, surely you can.
Wilfred Trotter (1872–1939)
Quoted in *Lancet*, 2:1340, 1965

5 Dr. Snow gave that blessed Chloroform & the effect was soothing, quieting & delightful beyond measure.
Victoria (1819–1901) Queen of England.
Journal
Describing her labour

ANATOMY

1 Anatomy is to physiology as geography to history; it describes the theatre of events.
Jean Fernel (1497–1558)
On the Natural Part of Medicine, Ch. 1

2 We anatomists are like the porters in Paris, who are acquainted with the narrowest and most distant streets, but who know nothing of what takes place in the houses!
Bernard Le Bovier de Fontenelle (1657–1757) French philosopher.
Attrib.

3 Anatomy is destiny.
Sigmund Freud (1856–1939) Austrian psychoanalyst.

4 You will have to learn many tedious things, . . . which you will forget the moment you have passed your final examination, but in anatomy it is better to have learned and lost than never to have learned at all.
W. Somerset Maugham (1874–1965) British writer and doctor.
Of Human Bondage, Ch. 54
Advice to first-year medical students

5 Surgeons and anatomists see no beautiful women in all their lives, but only a ghastly stack of bones with Latin names to them, and a network of nerves and muscles and tissues inflamed by disease.
Mark Twain (Samuel L. Clemens; 1835–1910) US writer.
Letter to the *Alta Californian*, San Francisco, 28 May 1867

ANOREXIA

1 Whether male or female, patients who don't eat because they don't experience hunger as an appropriate desire have to be taught not only to let themselves eat but also to allow themselves to hunger.
Sandra Gilbert
Womansize (Kim Chernin)

2 She didn't fear death itself, welcoming release from her long struggle between mind and body.
Mary Jane Moffat and Charlotte Painter
Describing an anorexic patient
Womansize (Kim Chernin)

ANTISEPTICS

1 Since the antiseptic treatment has been brought into full operation, and wounds and abscesses no longer poison the atmosphere with putrid exhalations, my wards, though in other respects under precisely the same circumstances as before, have completely changed their character; so that during the last nine months not a single instance of pyaemia, hospital gangrene or erysipelas has occurred in them.

As there appears to be no doubt regarding the cause of this change, the importance of the fact can hardly be exaggerated.
Joseph, Lord Lister (1827–1912) British surgeon.
British Medical Journal, 2:246, 1867

2   Soap and water and common sense are the best disinfectants.
Sir William Osler (1849–1919) Canadian physician.
Sir William Osler: Aphorisms, Ch. 5 (William B. Bean)

ANXIETY

1   But Jesus, when you don't have any money, the problem is food. When you have money, it's sex. When you have both, it's health, you worry about getting ruptured or something. If everything is simply jake then you're frightened of death.
J. P. Donleavy (1926–   ) US writer.

ASTHMA

1   Asthma is a disease that has practically the same symptoms as passion except that with asthma it lasts longer.
Anonymous

B

BABIES
See also **BIRTH, CHILDCARE, CHILDREN.**

1 There is no finer investment for any community than putting milk into babies.
Winston Churchill (1874–1965) British statesman.
Radio broadcast, 21 Mar 1943

2 Every baby born into the world is a finer one than the last.
Charles Dickens (1812–70) British novelist.
Nicholas Nickleby, Ch. 36

3 A loud noise at one end and no sense of responsibility at the other.
Ronald Knox (1888–1957) British Roman Catholic priest.
Attrib.

BALDNESS

1 The most delightful advantage of being bald—one can *hear* snowflakes.
R. G. Daniels (1916–) British magistrate.
The Observer, 'Sayings of the Week', 11 July 1976

2 A hair in the head is worth two in the brush.
Oliver Herford (1863–1935)

3 There's one thing about baldness – it's neat.
Don Herold
Attrib.

4 There is more felicity on the far side of baldness than young men can possibly imagine.
Logan Pearsall Smith (1865–1946) US-born British writer.
Afterthoughts, 2

BIORHYTHMS

1 I must consider more closely this cycle of good and bad days which I find coursing within myself. Passion, attachment, the urge to action, inventiveness, performance, order all alternate and keep their orbit; cheerfulness, vigor, energy, flexibility and fatigue, serenity as well as desire. Nothing disturbs the

cycle for I lead a simple life, but I must still find the time and order in
which I rotate.
Johann Wolfgang von Goethe (1749–1832) German poet and dramatist.
The Encyclopedia of Alternative Medicine and Self-Help (ed. Malcolm Hulke)

BIRTH
See also **PREGNANCY.**

1   Mary had a little lamb. The doctor fainted.
Anonymous

2   It is as natural to die as to be born; and to a little infant, perhaps, the one is
as painful as the other.
Sir Francis Bacon (1561–1626) English philosopher, lawyer, and politician.
Essays, 'Of Death'

3   Unto the woman he said, I will greatly multiply thy sorrow and thy conception; in sorrow thou shalt bring forth children.
Bible: Genesis
3:16

4   A woman when she is in travail hath sorrow, because her hour is come: but
as soon as she is delivered of the child, she remembereth no more the
anguish, for joy that a man is born into the world.
Bible: John
16:21

5   For all men have one entrance into life, and the like going out.
Bible: Wisdom
7:6

6   My mother groan'd, my father wept,
Into the dangerous world I leapt;
Helpless, naked, piping loud,
Like a fiend hid in a cloud.
William Blake (1757–1827) British poet.
Songs of Experience, 'Infant Sorrow'

7   Parturition is a physiological process – the same in the countess and in the
cow.
W. W. Chipman (1866–1950)

8   If men had to have babies they would only ever have one each.
Diana, Princess of Wales (1961–) Wife of Prince Charles.
The Observer, 'Sayings of the Week', 29 July 1984

9   It is not ultimately a matter of High Tech versus natural childbirth. The doctor does not necessarily always know best. A woman having a baby is doing
what she was designed for and that equips her with a kind of knowing. Surely
humility and respect on both sides is what is needed . . . The awareness of the

paper-thin divide between life and death can be life-enhancing or can shake
your confidence completely.
Mary Ellis
British Medical Journal, 25 Jan 1986

10 What they say of us is that we have a peaceful time
Living at home, while they do the fighting in war.
How wrong they are! I would very much rather stand
Three times in the front of battle than bear one child.
Euripides (484 BC–406 BC) Greek tragic dramatist.
Medea, 248

11 A man is not completely born until he be dead.
Benjamin Franklin (1706–90) US scientist and statesman.
Letters to Miss Hubbard

12 Man always dies before he is fully born.
Erich Fromm (1900–80) US psychologist and philosopher.
Man for Himself, Ch. 3

13 Man's main task in life is to give *birth* to himself.
Erich Fromm
Man for Himself, Ch. 4

14 If Nature had arranged that husbands and wives should have children alterna-
tively, there would never be more than *three* in a family.
Laurence Housman (1865–1959)

15 Birth may be a matter of a moment. But it is a unique one.
Frédérick Leboyer (1918–) French obstetrician.
Birth Without Violence

16 At the moment of childbirth, every woman has the same aura of isolation, as
though she were abandoned, alone.
Boris Pasternak (1890–1950) Russian writer.
Doctor Zhivago, Ch. 9, Sect. 3

17 There is nothing encourageth a woman sooner to be barren than hard travail
in child bearing.
Pliny the Elder (Gaius Plinius Secundus; 23 AD–79 AD) Roman writer.
Natural History

18 MACBETH. I bear a charmed life, which must not yield
To one of woman born.
MACDUFF. Despair thy charm;
And let the angel whom thou still hast serv'd
Tell thee Macduff was from his mother's womb
Untimely ripp'd.
William Shakespeare (1564–1616) English dramatist and poet.
Macbeth, V:8

19 A man may sympathize with a woman in childbed, though it is impossible that he should conceive himself as suffering her pains in his own proper person and character.
Adam Smith (1723–90) Scottish economist.
The Theory of Moral Sentiments, Pt. VII

20 Every moment dies a man,
Every moment one is born.
Alfred, Lord Tennyson (1809–92) British poet.
The Vision of Sin, Pt. IV

21 The explanation is quite simple. I wished to be near my mother.
James Whistler (1834–1903) US painter.
Attrib.
Explaining why he had been born in such an unfashionable place as Lowell, Massachusetts

22 Whither is fled the visionary gleam?
Where is it now, the glory and the dream?
Our birth is but a sleep and a forgetting.
William Wordsworth (1770–1850) British poet.
Ode: Intimations of Immortality

BIRTH CONTROL
See **CONTRACEPTION.**

BLINDNESS
See also **DISABILITY.**

1 . . . for three years I have been deprived of my sight. I wish you to learn from my own hand that thanks to the Divine Goodness I have recovered it. I see but as one sees after an operation, that is to say very dimly. Even this is a blessing for one who has had the misfortune to become blind. When I was sightless I cared for nothing, now I want to see everything .
Rosalba Carriera (1675–1757)
Letter, 23 Aug 1749

2 My soul is full of whispered song;
My blindness is my sight;
The shadows that I feared so long
Are all alive with light.
Alice Cary (1820–71)
Dying Hymn

3   It is not miserable to be blind; it is miserable to be incapable of enduring
    blindness.
    John Milton (1608–74) English poet.

4   Doth God exact day-labour, light deny'd,
    I fondly ask.
    John Milton
    Sonnet, 'When I Consider How my Light is Spent'

5   Why, in truth, should I not bear gently the deprivation of sight, when I may
    hope that it is not so much lost as revoked and retracted inwards, for the
    sharpening rather than the blunting of my mental edge?
    John Milton
    The Familiar Letters, No. 21, 24 Mar 1656

6   I have only one eye – I have a right to be blind sometimes.
    Horatio, Lord Nelson (1758–1805) English naval commander.
    Life of Nelson, Ch. 7 (Robert Southey)
    Nelson put his telescope to his blind eye to ignore the signal for his squadron
    to retreat at the Battle of Copenhagen

7   And so I betake myself to that course, which is almost as much as to see my-
    self go into the grave: for which, and all the discomforts that will accompany
    my being blind, the good God prepare me!
    Samuel Pepys (1633–1703) English diarist.
    Diary, 31 May 1669
    The last entry in his diary. Believing that he was going blind, Pepys aban-
    doned his diary, although he kept his sight for the rest of his life

8   There are none so blind as those who won't see.
    Proverb

9   Men are blind in their own cause.
    Proverb

10 In the Country of the Blind, the One-eyed Man is King.
    H. G. Wells (1866–1946) British writer.
    The Country of the Blind

BLOOD

1   Nurse, it was I who discovered that leeches have red blood.
    Baron Georges Cuvier (1769–1832) French zoologist.
    The Oxford Book of Death (D. Enright)
    On his deathbed when the nurse came to apply leeches

BODY
    See also **MIND AND BODY.**

1   A healthy body is the guest-chamber of the soul, a sick, its prison.
    Sir Francis Bacon (1561–1626) English philosopher, lawyer, and politician.
    Augmentis Scientiarum, 'Valetudo'

2   DIAPHRAGM, n. A muscular partition separating disorders of the chest from
    disorders of the bowels.
    Ambrose Bierce (1842–c. 1914) US writer and journalist.
    The Devil's Dictionary

3   The body is truly the garment of the soul, which has a living voice; for that
    reason it is fitting that the body simultaneously with the soul repeatedly sing
    praises to God through the voice.
    Hildegarde von Bingen (1098–1179)
    Letter to the Prelates of Mainz, c. 1178

4   It seems to me . . . highly dishonourable for a Reasonable Soul to live in so
    Divinely built a Mansion, as the Body she resides in, altogether unacquainted
    with the exquisite Structure of it.
    Robert Boyle (1627–91) Irish scientist.
    The Usefulness of Natural Philosophy, Pt. I

5   Of all these questions the one he asks most insistently is about man. How
    does he walk? How does the heart pump blood? What happens when he
    yawns and sneezes? How does a child live in the womb? Why does he die of
    old age? Leonardo discovered a centenarian in a hospital in Florence and
    waited gleefully for his demise so that he could examine his veins.
    Sir Kenneth Clark (1903–83) British historian.
    Civilisation
    Referring to Leonardo da Vinci

6   It's a burden to us even to be human beings—men with our own real body
    and blood; we are ashamed of it, we think it a disgrace and try to contrive to
    be some sort of impossible generalized man.
    Fyodor Mikhailovich Dostoevsky (1821–81) Russian writer.
    Notes from Underground, 2

7   We tolerate shapes in human beings that would horrify us if we saw them in
    a horse.
    W. R. Inge (1860–1954) British churchman and writer.
    Attrib.

8   The human body . . . indeed is like a ship; its bones being the stiff standing-
    rigging, and the sinews the small running ropes, that manage all the motions.
    Herman Melville (1819–91) US novelist.
    Redburn, Ch. 13

9   The human body is a machine which winds its own springs: the living image
    of perpetual movement.
    Julien Offroy de la Mettrie (1709–51)
    L'Homme machine

10 The abdomen is the reason why man does not easily take himself for a god.
    Friedrich Nietzsche (1844–1900) German philosopher.
    Beyond Good and Evil, 141

11 There is more wisdom in your body than in your deepest philosophy.
    Friedrich Nietzsche
    Human, All Too Human, Pt. II

12 It is in moments of illness that we are compelled to recognize that we live
    not alone but chained to a creature of a different kingdom, whole worlds
    apart, who has no knowledge of us and by whom it is impossible to make
    ourselves understood: our body.
    Marcel Proust (1871–1922) French writer.
    A la recherche du temps perdu: Le Côté de Guermantes

13 The body is not a permanent dwelling, but a sort of inn (with a brief sojourn
    at that) which is to be left behind when one perceives that one is a burden
    to the host.
    Seneca (c. 4 BC–65 AD) Roman writer.
    Epistulae ad Lucilium, CXX

14 If any thing is sacred the human body is sacred.
    Walt Whitman (1819–92) US poet.
    I Sing the Body Electric, 8

15 The human body is the best picture of the human soul.
    Ludwig Wittgenstein (1889–1951) Austrian philosopher.
    Philosophical Investigations

BRAIN
See also **MIND, MIND AND BODY.**

1 My brain: it's my second favourite organ.
   Woody Allen (Allen Stewart Konigsberg; 1935–) US film actor and director.
   Sleeper

2 BRAIN, n. An apparatus with which we think that we think.
   Ambrose Bierce (1842–c. 1914) US writer and journalist.
   The Devil's Dictionary

3 The brain is not an organ to be relied upon. It is developing monstrously. It
   is swelling like a goitre.
   Aleksandr Blok (1880–1921) Russian poet.

4 As long as our brain is a mystery, the universe, the reflection of the structure
   of the brain, will also be a mystery.
   Santiago Ramón y Cajal (1852–1934)
   Charlas de Café

5 We know the human brain is a device to keep the ears from grating on one another.
Peter de Vries (1910–) US writer.
Comfort Me with Apples, Ch. 1

6 The brain is a wonderful organ. It starts working the moment you get up in the morning, and does not stop until you get into the office.
Robert Frost (1875–1963) US poet.
Attrib.
Sometimes quoted as '. . . until you get up to make a speech'

7 And the mind must sweat a poison
. . . that, discharged not thence
Gangrenes the vital sense
And makes disorder true.
It is certain we shall attain
No life till we stamp on all
Life the tetragonal
Pure symmetry of the brain.
C. Day Lewis (1904–72) British poet.
Collected Poems 1929–1933

8 The brain has muscles for thinking as the legs have muscles for walking.
Julien Offroy de la Mettrie (1709–51)
L'Homme machine

9 It is good to rub and polish our brain against that of others.
Michel de Montaigne (1533–92) French essayist and moralist.
Essays, Bk. I

10 The brain is the organ of longevity.
George Alban Sacher (1917–)
Perspectives in Experimental Gerontology

11 If it is for mind that we are searching the brain, then we are supposing the brain to be much more than a telephone-exchange. We are supposing it to be a telephone-exchange along with subscribers as well.
Charles Scott Sherrington (1857–1952) British physiologist.
Man on his Nature

C

CANCER

1   Cancer's a Funny Thing:
    I wish I had the voice of Homer
    To sing of rectal carcinoma,
    Which kills a lot more chaps, in fact,
    Than were bumped off when Troy was sacked . . .
    J. B. S. Haldane (1892–1964) British geneticist.
    JBS (Ronald Clark)
    Written while mortally ill with cancer

2   While there are several chronic diseases more destructive to life than cancer,
    none is more feared.
    Charles H. Mayo (1865–1939) US physician.
    Annals of Surgery, 83:357, 1926

3   A typical triumph of modern science to find the only part of Randolph that
    was not malignant and remove it.
    Evelyn Waugh (1903–66) British novelist.
    Attrib.
    Referring to a report that Randolph Churchill had had a growth removed,
    but that it was not malignant

CASE HISTORY

1   A doctor who cannot take a good history and a patient who cannot give one
    are in danger of giving and receiving bad treatment.
    Anonymous
    Clues in the Diagnosis and Treatment of Heart Diseases, Introduction (Paul Dudley White)

2   The deficiencies which I think good to note . . . I will enumerate . . . . The
    first is the discontinuance of the ancient and serious diligence of Hippocrates,
    which used to set down a narrative of the special cases of his patients, and
    how they proceeded, and how they were judged by recovery or death.
    Sir Francis Bacon (1561–1626) English philosopher, lawyer, and politician.
    The Advancement of Learning, Bk. II

CHARITY

1 Private patients, if they do not like me, can go elsewhere; but the poor devils in the hospital I am bound to take care of.
John Abernethy (1764–1831) English surgeon.
Memoirs of John Abernethy, Ch. 5 (George Macilwain)

2 In medicine, charity offers to the poor the gains in medical skill, not the leavings.
Alan Gregg (1890–1957)
The Bampton Lectures

3 Sometimes give your services for nothing. . . . And if there be an opportunity of serving one who is a stranger in financial straits, give full assistance to all such. For where there is love of man, there is also love of the art.
Hippocrates (c. 460 BC–c. 377 BC) Greek physician.
Precepts, Sect. VI

4 Of gold she would not wear so much as a seal-ring, choosing to store her money in the stomachs of the poor rather than to keep it at her own disposal.
St. Jerome (c. 347–c. 420) Italian monk and scholar.
Letter CXXVII

5 The house which is not opened for charity will be opened to the physician.
The Talmud

CHILDBIRTH
See **BIRTH.**

CHILD CARE
See also **CHILDREN.**

1 If you take away a sick Child from its Parent or Nurse you break its Heart immediately: also, if there must be a Nurse to each Child what kind of an Hospital must there be to contain any Number of them . . . Add to all this it very seldom happens that a Mother can conveniently leave the Rest of her Family to go into an Hospital to attend her sick infant.
George Armstrong (d. 1781)

2 You can do anything with children if you only play with them.
Prince Otto von Bismarck (1815–98) German statesman.
Attrib.

3 Parents are the last people on earth who ought to have children.
Samuel Butler (1835–1902) British writer.
Notebooks

4   Children, in general, are overclothed and overfed. To these causes, I impute
    most of their diseases.
    William Cadogan (1711–97)
    Essays upon Nursing and Management of Children

5   Go to any village: The number of children born to most peasant families is
    ten, twelve, often as many as twenty. Yet only one, two or maybe four of
    these are living. Reduce the mortality rate, consult doctors, do something
    about the care of young children . . . They run about naked in their shifts in
    the snow and ice. Those who survive are healthy, but nineteen out of twenty
    die, *and what a loss to the state.*
    Catherine II (1729–96) Empress of Russia.
    Catherine the Great, Ch. 35 (Zoë Oldenbourg)

6   There is no finer investment for any community than putting milk into
    babies.
    Winston Churchill (1874–1965) British statesman.
    Radio broadcast, 21 Mar 1943

7   Infants do not cry without some legitimate cause.
    Ferrarius (16th century)
    The Advancement of Child Health (A. V. Neale)

8   The mother-child relationship is paradoxical and, in a sense, tragic. It re-
    quires the most intense love on the mother's side, yet this very love must
    help the child grow away from the mother and to become fully independent.
    Erich Fromm (1900–80) US psychologist and philosopher.

9   You may give them your love but not your thoughts.
    For they have their own thoughts.
    You may house their bodies but not their souls,
    For their souls dwell in the house of tomorrow, which you cannot visit, not
    even in your dreams.
    Kahlil Gibran (1883–1931) Lebanese mystic and poet.
    The Prophet, 'On Children'

10 God could not be everywhere and therefore he made mothers.
    Jewish proverb

11 At every step the child should be allowed to meet the real experiences of life;
    the thorns should never be plucked from his roses.
    Ellen Key (Karolina Sofia Key; 1849–1926) Swedish writer.
    The Century of the Child, Ch. 3

12 It is . . . sometimes easier to head an institute for the study of child guidance
    than it is to turn one brat into a decent human being.
    Joseph Wood Krutch (1893–1970) US essayist, critic, and teacher.
    If You Don't Mind My Saying, 'Whom Do We Picket Tonight?'

13 Children do not give up their innate imagination, curiosity, dreaminess easily. You have to love them to get them to do that.
R. D. Laing (1927–) British psychiatrist.
The Politics of Experience, Ch. 3

14 Slepe is the nourishment and food of a sucking child.
Thomas Phaer (c. 1510–60)
The Boke of Chyldren

15 But at three, four, five, and even six years the childish nature will require sports; now is the time to get rid of self-will in him, punishing him, but not so as to disgrace him.
Plato (c. 427 BC–347 BC) Greek philosopher.
Laws, VII, 794

CHILDREN
See also **CHILD CARE.**

1 One of the most obvious facts about grown-ups to a child is that they have forgotten what it is like to be a child.
Randall Jarrell (1914–65) US author.
Third Book of Criticism

2 Parents learn a lot from their children about coping with life.
Muriel Spark (1918–) British novelist.
The Comforters, Ch. 6

3 There are only two things a child will share willingly – communicable diseases and his mother's age.
Benjamin Spock (1903–) US pediatrician and psychiatrist.
Bartlett's Unfamiliar Quotations (Leonard Louis Levinson)

CHRISTIAN SCIENCE

1 Then comes the question, how do drugs, hygiene and animal magnetism heal? It may be affirmed that they do not heal, but only relieve suffering temporarily, exchanging one disease for another.
Mary Baker Eddy (1821–1910) US religious leader.
Science and Health, with Key to the Scriptures

2 Disease can carry its ill-effects no farther than mortal mind maps out the way . . . . Disease is an image of thought externalized . . . . We classify disease as error, which nothing but Truth or Mind can heal . . . . Disease is an experience of so-called mortal mind. It is fear made manifest on the body.
Mary Baker Eddy
Science and Health, with Key to the Scriptures

CIRCUMCISION

1   Ye shall circumcise the flesh of your foreskin; and it shall be a token of the covenant betwixt me and you.
Bible: Genesis
17:11

2   When they circumcised Herbert Samuel, they threw away the wrong bit.
David Lloyd George (1863–1945) British Liberal statesman.
Attrib., *The Listener*, 7 Sept 1978
Referring to the Liberal politician.

CLEANLINESS
See **HYGIENE.**

COLDS
See **COUGHS AND COLDS.**

CONCEPTION

1   Man is developed from an ovule, about the 1/25th of an inch in diameter, which differs in no respect from the ovules of other animals.
Charles Darwin (1809–82) British life scientist.
The Descent of Man, Ch. 1

2   A million million spermatozoa,
All of them alive:
Out of their cataclysm but one poor Noah
Dare hope to survive.
Aldous Huxley (1894–1964) British writer.
Fifth Philosopher's Song

3   Never neglect the history of a missed menstrual period.
Rutherford Morrison (1853–1939)
The Practitioner, Oct 1965

4   It's all any reasonable child can expect if the dad is present at the conception.
Joe Orton (1933–67) British dramatist.
Entertaining Mr. Sloane, III

CONSTIPATION

1 I have finally kum to the konklusion, that a good reliable sett ov bowels iz
   wurth more tu a man, than enny quantity ov brains.
   Henry Wheeler Shaw ('Josh Billings'; 1818–85)
   Josh Billings: His Sayings, Ch. 29

CONSULTANTS
See also **ANATOMY, DOCTORS, GENERAL PRACTITIONERS, SUR-
GEONS.**

1 An internist is someone who knows everything and does nothing.
   A surgeon is someone who does everything and knows nothing.
   A psychiatrist is someone who knows nothing and does nothing.
   A pathologist is someone who knows everything and does everything too late.
   Anonymous

2 Nouns of multitude (e.g., a pair of shoes, a gaggle of geese, a pride of lions)
   . . . . a rash of dermatologists, a hive of allergists, a scrub of interns, a chest
   of phthisiologists, or, a giggle of nurses, a flood of urologists, a pile of
   proctologists, an eyeful of ophthalmologists; or, a whiff of anesthesiologists, a
   staff of bacteriologists, a cast of orthopedic rheumatologists, a gargle of
   laryngologists.
   Anonymous
   Journal of the American Medical Association, 190:392, 1964

3 Choose your specialist and you choose your disease.
   Anonymous
   The Westminster Review, 18 May 1906

4 Patients consult so-called authorities. And I have become one also. Yet, we
   don't know more than the others. We are only the prey of hypochondriacs.
   August Bier (1861–1949)
   Aphorism

5 A medical chest specialist is long-winded about the short-winded.
   Kenneth T. Bird (1917–)

6 An expert is one who knows more and more about less and less.
   Nicholas Murray Butler (1862–1947)
   Commencement address, Columbia University

7 The specialist is a man who fears the other subjects.
   Martin H. Fischer (1879–1962)
   Fischerisms (Howard Fabing and Ray Marr)

8 Consultant specialists are a degree more remote (like bishops!); and therefore

(again like bishops) they need a double dose of Grace to keep them sensitive
to the personal and the pastoral.
Geoffrey Fisher, Archbishop of Canterbury (1887–1972) British churchman.
Lancet, 2:775, 1949

9   The consultant's first obligation is to the patient, not to his brother
    physician.
    Burton J. Hendrick (1870–1949)

10 One who limits himself to his chosen mode of ignorance.
    Elbert Hubbard (1856–1915) US writer and editor.

11 Specialist – A man who knows more and more about less and less.
    William J. Mayo (1861–1934) US surgeon.
    Also attributed to Nicholas Butler

12 Given one well-trained physician of the highest type he will do better work
    for a thousand people than ten specialists.
    William J. Mayo

13 Pediatricians eat because children don't.
    Meyer A. Perlstein (1902–   )

14 No man can be a pure specialist without being in the strict sense an idiot.
    George Bernard Shaw (1856–1950) Irish dramatist and critic.

CONTRACEPTION

1   I want to tell you a terrific story about oral contraception. I asked this girl to
    sleep with me and she said 'no'.
    Woody Allen (Allen Stewart Konigsberg; 1935–   ) US film actor and director.
    Woody Allen: Clown Prince of American Humor, Ch. 2, (Adler and Feinman)

2   The best contraceptive is a glass of cold water: not before or after, but
    instead.
    Anonymous
    Delegate at International Planned Parenthood Federation Conference.

3   Accidents will occur in the best-regulated families.
    Charles Dickens (1812–70) British novelist.
    David Copperfield, Ch. 28

4   The command 'Be fruitful and multiply' was promulgated according to our au-
    thorities, when the population of the world consisted of two people.
    W. R. Inge (1860–1954) British churchman and writer.
    More Lay Thoughts of a Dean

5   Where are the children I might have had? You may suppose I might have

wanted them. Drowned to the accompaniment of the rattling of a thousand douche bags.
Malcolm Lowry (1909–57) British novelist.
Under the Volcano, Ch. 10

6   It is now quite lawful for a Catholic woman to avoid pregnancy by a resort to mathematics, though she is still forbidden to resort to physics and chemistry.
H. L. Mencken (1880–1956) US journalist.
Notebooks, 'Minority Report'

7   Contraceptives should be used on every conceivable occasion.
Spike Milligan (1918–) British comic actor and writer.
The Last Goon Show of All

8   We want far better reasons for having children than not knowing how to prevent them.
Dora Russell (1894–1986)
Hypatia, Ch. 4

9   Skullion had little use for contraceptives at the best of times. Unnatural, he called them, and placed them in the lower social category of things along with elastic-sided boots and made-up bow ties. Not the sort of attire for a gentleman.
Tom Sharpe (1928–) British novelist.
Porterhouse Blue, Ch. 9

10 Protestant women may take the Pill. Roman Catholic women must keep taking the *Tablet*.
Irene Thomas (1920–) British writer.
Attrib.
The *Tablet* is a British Roman Catholic periodical

11 Marriages are not normally made to avoid having children.
Rudolf Virchow (1821–1902) German pathologist.
Bulletin of the New York Academy of Medicine, 4:995, 1928 (F. H. Garrison)

CONVALESCENCE

1   For Lawrence, existence was one continuous convalescence; it was as though he was newly reborn from a mortal illness every day of his life. What these convalescent eyes saw, his most casual speech would reveal.
Aldous Huxley (1894–1964) British writer.
The Olive Tree, 'D. H. Lawrence'

2   I enjoy convalescence. It is the part that makes the illness worth while.
George Bernard Shaw (1856–1950) Irish dramatist and critic.
Back to Methuselah, Pt. II

COUGHS AND COLDS

1   All who come my grave to see
    Avoid damp beds and think of me.
    Anonymous
    Epitaph of Lydia Eason, St Michael's, Stoke, England

2   Coughs and sneezes spread diseases.
    Anonymous
    Health slogan in the UK

3   Medicinal discovery,
    It moves in mighty leaps,
    It leapt straight past the common cold
    And gave it us for keeps.
    Pam Ayres British poet.
    Some of Me Poetry, 'Oh, No, I Got a Cold'

4   If you think that you have caught a cold, call in a good doctor. Call in three
    good doctors and play bridge.
    Robert Benchley (1889–1945) US humorist.
    From Bed to Worse, 'How to Avoid Colds'

5   'Ye can call it influenza if ye like', said Mrs. Machin. 'There was no influenza
    in my young days. We called a cold a cold'.
    Arnold Bennett (1867–1931) British novelist.
    The Card

6   The ancient Inhabitants of this Island were less troubled with Coughs when
    they went naked, and slept in Caves and Woods, than Men now in Cham-
    bers and Feather-beds.
    Sir Thomas Browne (1605–82) English physician and writer.
    A Letter to a Friend

7   A good gulp of hot whisky at bedtime – it's not very scientific, but it helps.
    Sir Alexander Fleming (1881–1955) British microbiologist.
    News summary, 22 Mar 1954
    When asked about a cure for colds

8   Cough: A convulsion of the lungs, vellicated by some sharp serosity.
    Samuel Johnson (1709–84) English lexicographer and writer.
    Dictionary of the English Language

9   A cough is something that you yourself can't help, but everybody else does
    on purpose just to torment you.
    Ogden Nash (1902–71) US poet.
    You Can't Get There from Here, 'Can I Get You a Glass of Water? or Please
    Close the Glottis After You'

10   Feed a cold and starve a fever.
     Proverb
     Commonly interpreted as meaning that one should eat with a cold but not
     with a fever. An alternative explanation is that if one 'feeds' a cold, by not
     taking care of it, one will end up having to deal with a fever.

11   Whiskey is the most popular of all the remedies that won't cure a cold.
     Jerry Vale
     Bartlett's Unfamiliar Quotations (Leonard Louis Levinson)

12   Saying 'Gesundheit' doesn't really help the common cold–but its about as
     good as anything the doctors have come up with.
     Earl Wilson
     Bartlett's Unfamiliar Quotations (Leonard Louis Levinson)

COUNSELLING

1   Advice is seldom welcome; and those who want it the most always like it the
    least.
    Earl of Chesterfield (1694–1773) English statesman.
    Letter to his son, 29 Jan 1748

2   One often calms one's grief by recounting it.
    Pierre Corneille (1606–84) French dramatist.
    Polyeucte, I:3

3   One stops being a child when one realizes that telling one's trouble does not
    make it better.
    Cesare Pavese (1908–50) Italian writer.
    The Business of Living: Diaries 1935–50

4   A trouble shared is a trouble halved.
    Proverb

5   It's queer how ready people always are with advice in any real or imaginary
    emergency, and no matter how many times experience has shown them to be
    wrong, they continue to set forth their opinions, as if they had received them
    from the Almighty!
    Annie Sullivan (1866–1936) US teacher of the handicapped.
    Letter, 12 June 1887

CURES
See also **DIAGNOSIS, HEALING, REMEDIES, TREATMENT.**

1   There is no curing a sick man who believes himself in health.
    Henri Amiel (1821–81) Swiss writer and philosopher.
    Journal, 6 Feb 1877

2   Cure the disease and kill the patient.
    Sir Francis Bacon (1561–1626) English philosopher, lawyer, and politician.
    Essays, 'Of Friendship'

3   There are no such things as incurable, there are only things for which man
    has not found a cure.
    Bernard Baruch (1870–1965) US financier and statesman.
    Speech, 30 Apr 1954; quoting his father, the surgeon Simon Baruch

4   Then Peter said, Silver and gold have I none; but such as I have give I thee:
    In the name of Jesus Christ of Nazareth rise up and walk.
    Bible: Acts
    3:6

5   And besought him that they might only touch the hem of his garment: and
    as many as touched were made perfectly whole.
    Bible: Matthew
    14:36

6   My father invented a cure for which there was no disease and unfortunately
    my mother caught it and died of it.
    Victor Borge (1909–   ) Danish-born US composer, actor, and musical
    comedian.
    In Concert

7   We all labour against our own cure, for death is the cure of all diseases.
    Sir Thomas Browne (1605–82) English physician and writer.
    Religio Medici

8   The Doctor fared even better. The fame of his new case spread far and wide.
    People seemed to think that if he could cure an elephant he could cure
    anything.
    Henry Cuyler Bunner (1855–96)
    Short Sixes, 'The Infidelity of Zenobia'

9   *Diseases* of their own Accord,
    But *Cures* come difficult and hard.
    Samuel Butler (1612–80) English poet and satirist.
    Satyr upon the Weakness and Misery of Man

10 Despair of all recovery spoils longevity,
    And makes men's miseries of alarming brevity.
    George Gordon, Lord Byron (1788–1824) British poet.
    Don Juan, II

11 A reckoning up of the cause often solves the malady.
    Celsus (25 BC–50 AD) Roman scholar.
    De Medicina, Prooemium

12 Medicine cures the man who is fated not to die.
    Chinese proverb

13 Physicians, when the cause of disease is discovered, consider that the cure is discovered.
Cicero (106 BC–43 BC) Roman orator and statesman.
Attrib.

14 When ill, indeed,
E'en dismissing the doctor don't *always* succeed.
George Colman, the Younger (1762–1836) British dramatist.
Lodgings for Single Gentlemen

15 What destroys one man preserves another.
Pierre Corneille (1606–84) French dramatist.
Cinna, II:1

16 You see—he's got a perfectly new idea. He never sees his patients. He's not interested in individuals, he prefers to treat a crowd. And he's organized these mass cures . . . And he cures thirty thousand people every Thursday.
Ruth Draper
Doctors and Diets

17 For extreme diseases, extreme methods of cure, as to restriction, are most suitable.
Hippocrates (c. 460 BC–c. 377 BC) Greek physician.
Aphorisms, 1

18 A good laugh and a long sleep are the best cures in the doctor's book.
Irish proverb

19 Is getting well ever an art
Or art a way to get well.
Robert Lowell (1917–77) US poet.
'Unwanted'

20 Gout is not relieved by a fine shoe nor a hangnail by a costly ring nor migraine by a tiara.
Plutarch (46 AD–120 AD) Greek biographer and essayist.
Moralia, 'Contentment'

21 The presence of the doctor is the beginning of the cure.
Proverb

22 Nothing hinders a cure so much as frequent change of medicine.
Seneca (c. 4 BC–65 AD) Roman writer.
Epistulae ad Lucilium

23 It is part of the cure to wish to be cured.
Seneca
Hippolytus, 249

24 They all thought she was dead; but my father he kept ladling gin down her throat till she came to so sudden that she bit the bowl off the spoon.
George Bernard Shaw (1856–1950) Irish dramatist and critic.
Pygmalion, III

25 There is only one cure for grey hair. It was invented by a Frenchman. It is called the guillotine.
P. G. Wodehouse (1881–1975) British-born US humorous writer.
The Old Reliable

D

DEAFNESS
See also **DISABILITY.**

1   There are two kinds of deafness. One is due to wax and is curable; the other
is not due to wax and is not curable.
Sir William Wilde (1815–76)

DEATH
See also **LIFE AND DEATH.**

1   I am dying with the help of too many physicians.
Alexander (III) the Great (356 BC–323 BC) King of Macedon.
Attrib.

2   Death is an acquired trait.
Woody Allen (Allen Stewart Konigsberg; 1935–   ) US film actor and director.
Woody Allen and His Comedy (E. Lax)

3   If your time ain't come not even a doctor can kill you.
American proverb

4   Death has got something to be said for it:
There's no need to get out of bed for it;
Wherever you may be,
They bring it to you, free.
Kingsley Amis (1922–   ) British writer.
'Delivery Guaranteed'

5   As Amr lay on his death-bed a friend said to him: 'You have often remarked
that you would like to find an intelligent man at the point of death, and to
ask him what his feelings were. Now I ask *you* that question. Amr replied, 'I
feel as if heaven lay close upon the earth and I between the two, breathing
through the eye of a needle.'
Amr Ibn Al-As (d. 664) Arab conqueror of Egypt.
The Harvest of a Quiet Eye (Alan L. Mackay)

6   Here lies the body of Mary Ann Lowder,
She burst while drinking a seidlitz powder;
Called from this world to her heavenly rest,
She should have waited till it effervesced.
Anonymous
Epitaph at Burlington, Massachusetts

7   Pain was my portion;

Physic was my food;
Groans my devotion;
Drugs did me no good.
Anonymous
Epitaph at Oldbury-on-Severn, England

8   There is a dignity in dying that doctors should not dare to deny.
Anonymous

9   Death must simply become the discreet but dignified exit of a peaceful person
from a helpful society that is not torn, not even overly upset by the idea of a
biological transition without significance, without pain or suffering, and ultimately without fear.
Philippe Ariès
The Hour of Our Death

10 I have often thought upon death, and I find it the least of all evils.
Sir Francis Bacon (1561–1626) English philosopher, lawyer, and politician.
An Essay on Death

11 I do not believe that any man fears to be dead, but only the stroke of death.
Sir Francis Bacon
An Essay on Death

12 It is natural to die as to be born; and to a little infant, perhaps, the one is as
painful as the other.
Sir Francis Bacon
Essays, 'Of Death'

13 Men fear Death as children fear to go in the dark, and as that natural fear in
children is increased with tales, so is the other.
Sir Francis Bacon
Essays, 'Of Death'

14 To die will be an awfully big adventure,
J. M. Barrie (1860–1937) Scottish dramatist and novelist.
Peter Pan, III

15 The physician cutteth off a long disease; and he that is today a king tomorrow shall die.
Bible: Ecclesiasticus
10:10

16 Man, that is born of a woman, hath but a short time to live.
Book of Common Prayer
'Burial of the Dead'

17 With what shift and pains we come into the World we remember not; but
'tis commonly found no easy matter to get out of it.
Sir Thomas Browne (1605–82) English physician and writer.
Christian Morals, Pt. II

18 I am not so much afraid of death, as ashamed thereof, 'tis the very disgrace
    and ignominy of our natures.
    Sir Thomas Browne
    Religio Medici

19 Since the order of the world is shaped by death, mightn't it be better for
    God if we refuse to believe in Him, and struggle with all our might against
    death without raising our eyes towards the heaven where He sits in silence?
    Albert Camus (1913–60) French existentialist writer.
    The Plague, II, Ch. 7

20 It is important what a man still plans at the end. It shows the measure of in-
    justice in his death.
    Elias Canetti (1905–   ) Bulgarian-born novelist.
    The Human Province

21 He had been, he said, a most unconscionable time dying; but he hoped that
    they would excuse it.
    Charles II (1630–85) King of England.
    History of England (Macaulay), Vol. I, Ch. 4
    On his deathbed

22 I am ready to meet my Maker. Whether my Maker is prepared for the ordeal
    of meeting me is another matter.
    Winston Churchill (1874–1965) British statesman.
    Said on his 75th birthday

23 Death . . . a friend that alone can bring the peace his treasures cannot pur-
    chase, and remove the pain his physicians cannot cure.
    Charles C. Colton (c. 1780–1832) British churchman and writer.
    Lacon, II, Ch. 110

24 Any man's death diminishes me, because I am involved in Mankinde;
    And therefore never send to know for whom the bell tolls;
    It tolls for thee.
    John Donne (1573–1631) English poet.
    Devotions, 17

25 So death, the most terrifying of ills, is nothing to us, since so long as we ex-
    ist, death is not with us; but when death comes, then we do not exist. It
    does not then concern either the living or the dead, since for the former it is
    not, and the latter are no more.
    Epicurus (341 BC–270 BC) Greek philosopher.
    Letter to Menoeceus

26 It hath been often said, that it is not death, but dying, which is terrible.
    Henry Fielding (1707–54) English novelist.
    Amelia, Bk. III, Ch. 4

27   In vain we shall penetrate more and more deeply the secrets of the structure
     of the human body, we shall not dupe nature; we shall die as usual.
     Bernard de Fontenelle (1657–1757) French philosopher.
     Dialogues des morts, Dialogue V

28   When he can keep life no longer in, he makes a fair and easie passage for it
     to go out.
     Thomas Fuller (1608–61) English historian.
     The Holy State, Ch. 17

29   The doctors found, when she was dead –
     Her last disorder mortal.
     Oliver Goldsmith (1728–74) Irish-born English writer.
     Elegy on Mrs. Mary Blaize

30   Grieve not that I die young. Is it not well
     To pass away ere life hath lost its brightness?
     Lady Flora Hastings (1806–39) British poet.
     Swan Song

31   Death is a delightful hiding-place for weary men.
     Herodotus (484 BC–424 BC) Greek historian.
     Histories, VII, 46

32   Death . . . It's the only thing we haven't succeeded in completely vulgarizing.
     Aldous Huxley (1894–1964) British writer.
     Eyeless in Gaza, Ch. 31

33   Ignore death until the last moment; then when it can't be ignored any longer
     have yourself squirted full of morphia and shuffle off in a corner.
     Aldous Huxley
     Time Must Have A Stop

34   You mean what everybody means nowadays . . . Ignore death up to the last
     moment; then, when it can't be ignored any longer, have yourself squirted
     full of morphia and shuffle off in a coma.
     Aldous Huxley
     Time Must Have a Stop

35   Death is the poor man's best physician.
     Irish proverb

36   Now more than ever seems it rich to die,
     To cease upon the midnight with no pain.
     John Keats (1795–1821) British poet.
     Ode to a Nightingale

37   A long illness seems to be placed between life and death, in order to make
     death a comfort both to those who die and to those who remain.
     Jean de La Bruyère (1645–96) French writer and moralist.
     Caractères, Ch. 11

38   Death defies the doctor.
Latin proverb

39   Death is better than disease.
Henry Wadsworth Longfellow (1807–82) US poet.
Christus: A Mystery, Pt. II, Sect. 1

40   There is . . . no death . . . There is only . . . *me* . . . *me* . . . *who is going to die* . . .
André Malraux (1901–76) French writer and statesman.
The Royal Way

41   It is the only disease you don't look forward to being cured of.
Herman J. Mankiewicz (1897–1953) US journalist and screenwriter.
Citizen Kane
Referring to death

42   'Dying', he said to me, 'is a very dull, dreary affair.' Suddenly he smiled. 'And my advice to you is to have nothing whatever to do with it,' he added.
W. Somerset Maugham (1874–1965) British writer and doctor.
Escape from the Shadows (Robin Maugham)
Said shortly before his death

43   Dying is the most hellishly boresome experience in the world! Particularly when it entails dying of 'natural causes'.
W. Somerset Maugham
The Two Worlds of Somerset Maugham, Ch. 22 (Wilmon Menard)

44   Whom the gods love dies young.
Menander (c. 341 BC–c. 290 BC) Greek dramatist.
Dis Exapaton

45   If it be a short and violent death, we have no leisure to fear it; if otherwise, I perceive that according as I engage myself in sickness, I do naturally fall into some disdain and contempt of life.
Michel de Montaigne (1533–92) French essayist and moralist.
Essays

46   Who was it that said the living are the dead on holiday?
Terry Nation
Dr. Who, BBC TV, 1980

47   Die, my dear doctor! That's the last thing I shall do!
Lord Palmerston (1784–1865) British statesman.
Last words

48   Many men on the point of an edifying death would be furious if they were suddenly restored to life.
Cesare Pavese (1908–50) Italian writer.

49   When a man lies dying, he does not die from the disease alone. He dies from
     his whole life.
     Charles Péguy (1873–1914) French writer.
     Basic Verities, 'The Search for Truth'

50   If your time hasn't come not even a doctor can kill you.
     Meyer A. Perlstein (1902–)

51   Dying
     is an art, like everything else.
     I do it exceptionally well.
     Sylvia Plath (1932–63) US writer.
     Lady Lazarus

52   He whom the gods love dies young, while he has his strength and senses and
     wits.
     Plautus (c. 254 BC–184 BC) Roman dramatist.
     Bacchides, IV:8

53   Here am I, dying of a hundred good symptoms.
     Alexander Pope (1688–1744) English poet.
     Anecdotes by and about Alexander Pope (Joseph Spence)

54   As soon as man is born he begins to die.
     Proverb

55   Death defies the doctor.
     Proverb

56   The first breath is the beginning of death.
     Proverb

57   Death is the greatest kick of all, that's why they save it for last.
     Robert Raisner
     Graffiti, 'Death'

58   He who pretends to look on death without fear lies. All men are afraid of dy-
     ing, this is the great law of sentient beings, without which the entire human
     species would soon be destroyed.
     Jean-Jacques Rousseau (1712–78) French philosopher.
     Julie, or the New Eloise

59   Death is the privilege of human nature,
     And life without it were not worth our taking.
     Nicholas Rowe (1674–1718) English dramatist.
     The Fair Penitent, V:1

60   Many people would sooner die than think. In fact they do.
     Bertrand Russell (1872–1970) British philosopher.
     Thinking about Thinking (A. Flew)

61   You will die not because you're ill, but because you're alive.
     Seneca (4 BC–65 AD) Roman writer.
     Epistulae ad Lucilium, LXXVII

62   He had rather
     Groan so in perpetuity, than be cured
     By the sure physician, death.
     William Shakespeare (1564–1616) English dramatist and poet.
     Cymbeline

63   By medicine life may be prolonged, yet death will seize the doctor too.
     William Shakespeare
     Cymbeline

64   CORNELIUS. The Queen is dead.
     CYMBELINE. Who worse than a physician
     Would this report become? But I consider
     By med'cine life may be prolong'd, yet death
     Will seize the doctor too.
     William Shakespeare
     Cymbeline, V:5

65   Why, he that cuts off twenty years of life
     Cuts off so many years of fearing death.
     William Shakespeare
     Julius Caesar, III:1

66   As flies to wanton boys are we to th' gods –
     They kill us for their sport.
     William Shakespeare
     King Lear, IV:1

67   After all, what *is* death? Just nature's way of telling us to slow down.
     Dick Sharples
     In Loving Memory, Yorkshire Television, 1979

68   Death must be distinguished from dying, with which it is often confused.
     Sydney Smith (1771–1845) British churchman, essayist, and wit.
     The Smith of Smiths (Pearson)

69   My name is DEATH; THE LAST BEST FRIEND AM I.
     Robert Southey (1774–1843) British poet.
     Carmen Nuptiale: the Lay of the Laureate, 'The Dream'

70   It is impossible that anything so natural, so necessary, and so universal as
     death, should ever have been designed by Providence as an evil to mankind.
     Jonathan Swift (1667–1745) Anglo-Irish priest, satirist and poet.
     'Thoughts on Religion'

71   Even so, in death the same unknown will appear as ever known to me. And
     because I love this life, I know I shall love death as well.

The child cries out when from the right breast the mother takes it away, in
the very next moment to find in the left one its consolation.
Rabindranath Tagore (1861–1941) Indian poet and philosopher.
Gitanjali

72   Do not go gentle into that good night,
     Old age should burn and rave at close of day;
     Rage, rage, against the dying of the light.
     Dylan Thomas (1914–53) Welsh poet.
     Do not go gentle into that good night

73   Death is the price paid by life for an enhancement of the complexity of a
     live organism's structure.
     Arnold Toynbee (1889–1975) British historian.
     Life After Death

74   The human race is the only one that knows it must die, and it knows this
     only through its experience. A child brought up alone and transported to a
     desert island would have no more idea of death than a cat or a plant.
     Voltaire (François-Marie Arouet; 1694–1778) French writer and philosopher.
     The Oxford Book of Death (D.J. Enright)

75   Man has given a false importance to death
     Any animal plant or man who dies
     adds to Nature's compost heap
     becomes the manure without which
     nothing could grow nothing could be created
     Death is simply part of the process.
     Peter Weiss (1916–82) German novelist and dramatist.
     Marat/Sade, I:12

76   One can survive everything nowadays, except death.
     Oscar Wilde (1854–1900) Irish writer and wit.
     A Woman of No Importance, I

77   The Doctor said that Death was but
     A scientific fact.
     Oscar Wilde
     The Ballad of Reading Gaol

78   I expect I shall have to die beyond my means.
     Oscar Wilde
     Accepting a glass of champagne on his deathbed

DENTISTS
See also **TEETH**.

1   Stranger! Approach this spot with gravity!

John Brown is filling his last cavity.
Epitaph of a dentist

DIABETES

1 Many a diabetic has stayed alive by stealing the bread denied him by his
   doctor.
   Martin H. Fischer (1879–1962)
   Fischerisms (Howard Fabing and Ray Marr)

DIAGNOSIS
See also **CURES, HEALING, REMEDIES, TREATMENT.**

1 To avoid delay, please have all your symptoms ready.
   Anonymous
   Notice in a doctor's waiting-room

2 The fingers should be kept on the pulse at least until the hundredth beat in
   order to judge of its kind and character; the friends standing round will be all
   the more impressed because of the delay, and the physician's words will be received with just that much more attention.
   Archimathaeus (c. 1100)
   The Coming of a Physician to his Patient

3 A smart mother makes often a better diagnosis than a poor doctor.
   August Bier (1861–1949)

4 It is more important to cure people than to make diagnoses.
   August Bier

5 DIAGNOSIS, n. A physician's forecast of disease by the patient's pulse and
   purse.
   Ambrose Bierce (1842–c. 1914) US writer and journalist.
   The Devil's Dictionary

6 Physicians must discover the weaknesses of the human mind, and even con-
   descend to humour them, or they will never be called in to cure the infirmities of the body.
   Charles C. Colton (1780–1832) British churchman and writer.
   Lacon, 1

7 In diagnosis think of the easy first.
   Martin H. Fischer (1879–1962)
   Fischerisms (Howard Fabing and Ray Marr)

8 There are men who would even be afraid to commit themselves to the doctrine that castor oil is a laxative.
   Camille Flammarion (1842–1925)

9   The doctor may also learn more about the illness from the way the patient
    tells the story than from the story itself.
    James B. Herrick (1861–1954)
    Memories of Eighty Years, Ch. 8

10 In acute diseases it is not quite safe to prognosticate either death or recovery.
    Hippocrates (c. 460 BC–c. 377 BC) Greek physician.
    Aphorisms, II

11 Declare the past, diagnose the present, foretell the future.
    Hippocrates
    Epidemics

12 The most important requirement of the art of healing is that no mistakes or
    neglect occur. There should be no doubt or confusion as to the application of
    the meaning of complexion and pulse. These are the maxims of the art of
    healing.
    Huang Ti (The Yellow Emperor; 2697 BC–1597 BC)
    Nei Ching Su Wên, Bk. 4, Sect. 13

13 Physicians think they do a lot for a patient when they give his disease a
    name.
    Immanuel Kant (1724–1804) German philosopher.
    Attrib.

14 We are too much accustomed to attribute to a single cause that which is the
    product of several, and the majority of our controversies come from that.
    Baron Justus von Liebig (1803–73) German chemist.
    Attrib.

15 The examining physician often hesitates to make the necessary examination
    because it involves soiling the finger.
    William J. Mayo (1861–1939) US surgeon.
    Journal-Lancet, 35:339, 1915

16 The fact that your patient gets well does not prove that your diagnosis was
    correct.
    Samuel J. Meltzer (1851–1921)
    Attrib.

17 There is no royal road to diagnosis.
    Robert Tuttle Morris (1857–1945)
    Doctors versus Folks, Ch. 4

18 The physician who is attending a patient . . . has to know the cause of the
    ailment before he can cure it.
    Mo-tze (fl. 5th–4th century BC)
    Ethical and Political Works, Bk. IV, Ch. 14

19 A disease known is half cured.
    Proverb

DIGESTION
See also **INDIGESTION.**

1   A good eater must be a good man; for a good eater must have a good diges-
    tion, and a good digestion depends upon a good conscience.
    Benjamin Disraeli (1804–81) British statesman.
    The Young Duke

2   I am convinced digestion is the great secret of life.
    Sydney Smith (1771–1845) English clergyman, essayist, and wit.
    Letters, to Arthur Kinglake

3   The fate of a nation has often depended upon the good or bad digestion of a
    prime minister.
    Voltaire (François-Marie Arouet; 1694–1778) French writer and philosopher.
    Bartlett's Unfamiliar Quotations (Leonard Louis Levinson)

DISABILITY

1   If there are any of you at the back who do not hear me, please don't raise
    your hands because I am also nearsighted.
    W. H. Auden (1907–73) British poet.
    The opening words of a lecture
    In *Book of the Month Club News*, Dec 1946

2   Another great Advantage of Deformity is, that it tends to the Improvement
    of the Mind. A man, that cannot shine in his Person, will have recourse to
    his Understanding: and attempt to adorn that Part of him, which alone is ca-
    pable of ornament.
    William Hay (1695–1755)
    Essay on Deformity

3   You are not crippled at all unless your mind is in a splint.
    Frank Scully
    Bartlett's Unfamiliar Quotations (Leonard Louis Levinson)

DISEASE
See also **ILLNESS, INCURABLE DISEASE.**

1   We are led to think of diseases as isolated disturbances in a healthy body, not
    as the phases of certain periods of bodily development.
    Sir Clifford Allbutt (1836–1925)
    Bulletin of the New York Academy of Medicine, 4:1000, 1928 (F.H. Garrison)

2   Disease is in essence the result of conflict between soul and mind–So long as
    our souls and personalities are in harmony all is joy and peace, happiness and
    health. It is when our personalities are led astray from the path laid down by

the soul, either by our own wordly desires or by the persuasion of others, that a conflict arises.
Dr. Edward Bach (1880–1936) British doctor; founder of Bach Flower Remedies.
The Alternative Health Guide (Brian Inglis and Ruth West)

4   Diseases . . . crucify the soul of man, attenuate our bodies, dry them, wither them, rivel them up like old apples, make them as so many Anatomies.
Robert Burton
The Anatomy of Melancholy, I

5   Disease is very old, and nothing about it has changed. It is we who change, as we learn to recognize what was formerly imperceptible.
Jean Martin Charcot (1825–93) French neurologist.
De l'expectation en médecine

6   Most of those evils we poor mortals know
From doctors and imagination flow.
Charles Churchill (1731–64) English poet.
The Prophecy of Famine

7   A bodily disease, which we look upon as whole and entire within itself, may, after all, be but a symptom of some ailment in the spiritual part.
Nathaniel Hawthorne (1804–64) US novelist and writer.
The Scarlet Letter, Ch. 10

8   Perfect health, like perfect beauty, is a rare thing; and so, it seems, is perfect disease.
Peter Mere Latham (1789–1875) US poet and essayist.
General Remarks on the Practice of Medicine, Ch. 10, Pt. ii

9   Disease makes men more physical, it leaves them nothing but body.
Thomas Mann (1875–1955) German novelist.
The Magic Mountain, 4

10 Fever the eternal reproach to the physicians.
John Milton (1608–74) English poet.
Paradise Lost, Bk. XI

11 Confront disease at its first stage.
Aulus Flaccus Persius (34 AD–62 AD) Roman satirist.
Satires, III

12 Medicine, to produce health, has to examine disease.
Plutarch (c. 46–c. 120) Greek biographer and essayist.
Lives, 'Demetrius', I

13 Diseases are the tax on pleasures.
    John Ray (1627–1705) English naturalist.
    English Proverbs

14 The diseases which destroy a man are no less natural than the instincts which
    preserve him.
    George Santayana (1863–1952) Spanish-born US philosopher, poet, and critic.
    Dialogues in Limbo, 3

15 Disease is not of the body but of the place.
    Seneca (c. 4 BC–65 AD) Roman writer.
    Epistulae ad Lucilium

16 Not even medicine can master incurable diseases.
    Seneca (c. 4 BC–65 AD) Roman writer.
    Epistulae ad Lucilium, XCIV

17 The development of industry has created many new sources of danger. Occu-
    pational diseases are socially different from other diseases, but not biologically.
    Henry E. Sigerist (1891–1957)
    Journal of the History of Medicine and Allied Sciences, 13:214, 1958

18 Disease creates poverty and poverty disease. The vicious circle is closed.
    Henry E. Sigerist (1891–1957) Swiss medical historian.
    Medicine and Human Welfare, Ch. 1

19 The man of the present day would far rather believe that disease is connected
    only with immediate causes for the fundamental tendency in the modern view
    of life is always to seek what is most convenient.
    Rudolf Steiner (1861–1925) Austrian philosopher, founder of anthroposophy.
    The Manifestations of Karma, Lecture III

DISSECTION

1 Her body dissected by fiendish men,
   Her bones anatomized,
   Her soul, we trust, has risen to God,
   Where few physicians rise.
   Anonymous
   Epitaph of Ruth Sprague

2 No man should marry until he has studied anatomy and dissected at least one
   woman.
   Honoré de Balzac (1799–1850) French novelist.
   The Physiology of Marriage, Meditation V, Aphorism 28

3 BODY-SNATCHER, n. A robber of grave-worms. One who supplies the

young physicians with that with which the old physicians have supplied the
undertaker.
Ambrose Bierce (1842–c. 1914) US writer and journalist.
The Devil's Dictionary

4   GRAVE, n. A place in which the dead are laid to await the coming of the
medical student.
Ambrose Bierce
The Devil's Dictionary

5   O speculator concerning this machine of ours let it not distress you that you
impart knowledge of it through another's death, but rejoice that our Creator
has ordained the intellect to such excellence of perception.
Leonardo da Vinci (1452–1519) Italian artist, architect, and engineer.
Quaderni d'Anatomia, Vol. II

DOCTORS

See also ANATOMY, CONSULTANTS, DOCTORS AND PATIENTS,
GENERAL PRACTITIONERS, MEDICAL STUDENTS, SURGEONS.

1   In illness the physician is a father; in convalescence a friend; when health is
restored, he is a guardian.
Anonymous
Brahmanic saying

2   These are the duties of a physician: First . . . to heal his mind and to give
help to himself before giving it to anyone else.
Anonymous
Epitaph of an Athenian doctor, 2 AD (*Journal of the American Medical Association*, 189:989, 1964)

3   One physician cures you of the colic; two physicians cure you of the
medicine.
Anonymous
Journal of the American Medical Association, 190:765, 1964 (Vincent J. Derbes)

4   Fifty years ago the successful doctor was said to need three things; a top hat
to give him Authority, a paunch to give him Dignity, and piles to give him
an Anxious Expression.
Anonymous
Lancet, 1:169, 1951

5   No one appreciates the medical profession more highly than myself. Doctors
are the most generous of men; but they are unwise when they represent doctoring either as an art or a science. . . . doctors would be better appreciated if
they would frankly admit that doctoring is like logic.
Anonymous
More from a Lawyer's Notebook, 'Doctors'

6   No man is a good physician who has never been sick.
    Arabic proverb

7   My dear old friend King George V always told me that he would never have
    died but for that vile doctor.
    Margot Asquith (1865–1945) Wife of Herbert Asquith.
    Referring to Lord Dawson of Penn

8   Give me a doctor partridge-plump,
    Short in the leg and broad in the rump,
    An endomorph with gentle hands
    Who'll never make absurd demands
    That I abandon all my vices
    Nor pull a long face in a crisis,
    But with a twinkle in his eye
    Will tell me that I have to die.
    W. H. Auden (1907–73) British poet.
    Nones, 'Footnotes to Dr. Sheldon'

9   Doctors and undertakers
    Fear epidemics of good health.
    Gerald Barzan

10 Honour a physician with the honour due unto him for the uses which ye may
    have of him: for the Lord hath created him.
    For of the most High cometh healing, and he shall receive honour of the
    king.
    Bible: Ecclesiasticus
    38:1–2

11 And he said unto them, Ye will surely say unto me this proverb, Physician,
    heal thyself: whatsoever we have heard done in Capernaum, do also here in
    thy country.
    Bible: Luke
    4:23

12 Medical scientists are nice people, but you should not let them treat you.
    August Bier (1861–1949)
    Attrib.

13 PHYSICIAN, n. One upon whom we set our hopes when ill and our dogs
    when well.
    Ambrose Bierce (1842–c. 1914) US writer and journalist.
    The Devil's Dictionary

14 Sagacity, manual dexterity, quiet reserve, a kind heart, and a conscience –
    these, if there at all, are always at hand, always inestimable; and if wanting,
    . . . I can profit my patient and myself nothing.
    John Brown (1810–82)
    Horae Subsecivae

15   A skilful leech is better far
     Than half a hundred men of war.
     Samuel Butler (1612–80) English satirist.
     Hudibras, Pt. I

16   How does one become a good doctor? . . . As I understand it a good doctor is
     one who is shrewd in diagnosis and wise treatment; but, more than that, he
     is a person who never spares himself in the interest of his patients; and in ad-
     dition he is a man who studies the patient not only as a case but also as an
     individual. . . . The good doctor, whether general practitioner or specialist, is
     also a man who studies the patient's personality as well as his disease.
     Sir Hugh Cairns (1896–1952)
     Lancet, 2:665, 1949

17   If the clinician, as observer, wishes to see things as they really are, he must
     make a *tabula rasa* of his mind and proceed without any preconceived notions
     whatever.
     Jean Martin Charcot (1825–93) French neurologist.

18   Doctors are just the same as lawyers; the only difference is that lawyers
     merely rob you, whereas doctors rob you and kill you, too.
     Anton Chekhov (1860–1904) Russian dramatist.
     Ivanov, I

19   The superior doctor prevents sickness;
     The mediocre doctor attends to impending sickness;
     The inferior doctor treats actual sickness.
     Chinese proverb

20   The trouble with doctors is not that they don't know enough, but that they
     don't see enough.
     Sir Dominic J. Corrigan (1802–80)

21   When a doctor does go wrong he is the first of criminals. He has nerve and
     he has knowledge.
     Arthur Conan Doyle (1856–1930) British writer and creator of Sherlock
     Holmes.
     The Speckled Band

22   'What sort of doctor is he?'
     'Oh, well, I don't known much about his ability; but he's got a very good
     bedside manner!'
     George du Maurier (1834–96) British novelist and cartoonist.
     Caption to cartoon, *Punch*, 15 Mar 1884

23   In the hands of the discoverer, medicine becomes a heroic art . . . wherever
     life is dear he is a demigod.
     Ralph Waldo Emerson (1803–82) US poet and essayist.
     Uncollected Lectures, 'Resources'

24 Half-informed physicians are generally skeptics.
    Baron Ernst von Feuchtersleben (1806–49)
    Dietetics of the Soul, XII

25 A doctor must work eighteen hours a day and seven days a week. If you cannot console yourself to this, get out of the profession.
    Martin H. Fischer (1879–1962)
    Fischerisms (Howard Fabing and Ray Marr)

26 Medicine is the one place where all the show is stripped of the human drama. You, as doctors, will be in a position to see the human race stark naked – not only physically, but mentally and morally as well.
    Martin H. Fischer
    Fischerisms (Wherry, Holmes, and Baehr)

27 Physicians, like beer, are best when they are old.
    Thomas Fuller (1608–61) English historian.
    The Holy State and the Profane State

28 The physician is Nature's assistant.
    Galen (fl. 2nd century) Greek physician.
    Commentary on Hippocrates' De Humoribus, Bk. I, Prooemium

29 That physician will hardly be thought very careful of the health of others who neglects his own.
    Galen
    Of Protecting the Health, Bk. V

30 See, one physician, like a sculler plies,
    The patient lingers and by inches dies,
    But two physicians, like a pair of oars
    Waft him more swiftly to the Stygian shores.
    Sir Samuel Garth (1661–1719)
    Attrib.

31 A physician ought to be extremely watchful against covetousness, for it is a vice imputed, justly or unjustly, to his Profession.
    Thomas Gisborne (1758–1846)
    The Duties of Physicians

32 It is so hard that one cannot really have confidence in doctors and yet cannot do without them.
    Johann Wolfgang von Goethe (1749–1832) German poet, dramatist, and scientist.

33 The crowd of physicians has killed me.
    Hadrian (Publius Aelius Hadrianus; 76 AD–138 AD) Roman emperor.
    Essays, Bk. II (Michel de Montaigne)

34 The people in this world put on a tremendous show, and doctors have a front
    row seat.
    Carl Augustus Hamann (1868–1930)
    Aphorism

35 Do not dwell in a city whose governor is a physician.
    Hebrew Proverb

36 A physician who is a lover of wisdom is the equal to a god.
    Hippocrates (c. 460 BC–c. 377 BC) Greek physician.
    Decorum, V

37 Foolish the doctor who despises the knowledge acquired by the ancients.
    Hippocrates
    Entering the World (M. Odent)

38 Some patients, though conscious that their condition is perilous, recover their
    health simply through their contentment with the goodness of the physician.
    Hippocrates
    Precepts, VI

39 A man of very moderate ability may be a good physician, if he devotes him-
    self faithfully to the work.
    Oliver Wendell Holmes (1809–94) US writer and humorist.
    Medical Essays, 'Scholastic and Bedside Teaching'

40 It is unnecessary – perhaps dangerous – in medicine to be too clever.
    Sir Robert Hutchison (1871–1960)
    Lancet, 2:61, 1938

41 I suppose one has a greater sense of intellectual degradation after an interview
    with a doctor than from any human experience.
    Alice James (1848–92) US diarist.
    The Diary of Alice James, 27 Sept 1890

42 Better go without medicine than call in an unskilful physician.
    Japanese proverb

43 It is incident to physicians, I am afraid, beyond all other men, to mistake
    subsequence for consequence.
    Samuel Johnson (1709–84) English lexicographer and writer.
    Life of Johnson (J. Boswell), Vol. I

44 Many funerals discredit a physician.
    Ben Jonson (1572–1637) English dramatist.

45 The doctors allow one to die, the charlatans kill.
    Jean de La Bruyère (1645–96) French writer and moralist.
    Caractères

46 As long as men are liable to die and are desirous to live, a physician will be made fun of, but he will be well paid.
Jean de La Bruyère
Caractères, 14

47 Though physician to others, yet himself full of sores.
Latin proverb

48 I often say a great doctor kills more people than a great general.
Baron Gottfried Wilhelm von Leibnitz (1646–1716) German philosopher and mathematician.

49 A doctor is a man licensed to make grave mistakes.
Leonard Louis Levinson
Bartlett's Unfamiliar Quotations (Leonard Louis Levinson)

50 But a doctor who has gone into lonely and discouraged homes, where there was fear for the sick, and no one else at hand to administer remedy, and give hope, can really say, 'I amount to something. I'm worth while.'
Carlton K. Matson (1890–1948)
The Cleveland Press

51 Mrs. Carey thought there were only four professions for a gentleman, the Army, the Navy, the Law, and the Church. She had added medicine . . . but did not forget that in her young days no one ever considered the doctor a gentleman.
W. Somerset Maugham (1874–1965) British writer and doctor.
Of Human Bondage, Ch. 33

52 As he approached the place where a meeting of doctors was being held, he saw some elegant limousines and remarked, 'The surgeons have arrived.' Then he saw some cheaper cars and said, 'The physicians are here, too.' A few scattered model-T Fords led him to infer that there were pathologists present. And when he saw a row of overshoes inside, under the hat rack, he is reported to have remarked, 'Ah, I see there are laboratory men here.'
William J. Mayo (1861–1939) US surgeon.
The Way of an Investigator, Ch. 19 (Walter B. Cannon)

53 Every idiot, priest, Jew, monk, actor, barber and old woman, fancy themselves physicians.
Medieval saying

54 English physicians kill you, the French let you die.
William Lamb, Lord Melbourne (1779–1848) British statesman.
Queen Victoria, Ch. 5 (Elizabeth Longford)

55 I wasn't driven into medicine by a social conscience but by rampant curiosity.
Jonathan Miller (1936–) British writer and doctor.

56   No doctor takes pleasure in the health even of his friends.
     Michel de Montaigne (1533–92) French essayist and moralist.
     Essays, I

57   Probably to no other are the strengths and weakness of humanity so completely laid bare.
     James G. Mumford (1863–1914)

58   You medical people will have more lives to answer for in the other world than even we generals.
     Napoleon 1 (Napoleon Bonaparte; 1769–1821) French Emperor.
     Napoleon in Exile (Barry O'Meara)

59   The most dangerous physicians are those who can act in perfect mimicry of the born physician.
     Friedrich Nietzsche (1844–1900) German philosopher.
     Human, All Too Human, Pt. II

60   All knowledge attains its ethical value and its human significance only by the humane sense in which it is employed. Only a good man can be a great physician.
     Hermann Nothnagel (1841–1905)

61   There are only two sorts of doctors: those who practise with their brains, and those who practise with their tongues.
     Sir William Osler (1849–1919) Canadian physician.
     Aequanimitas, with Other Addresses, 'Teaching and Thinking'

62   To prevent disease, to relieve suffering and to heal the sick – this is our work.
     Sir William Osler
     Aequanimitas, with Other Addresses, 'Chauvinism in Medicine'

63   A physician who treats himself has a fool for a patient.
     Sir William Osler
     Sir William Osler: Aphorisms, Ch. I (William B. Bean)

64   We doctors have always been a simple trusting folk. Did we not believe Galen implicitly for 1500 years and Hippocrates for more than 2000?
     Sir William Osler

65   God and the Doctor we alike adore
     But only when in danger, not before;
     The danger o'er, both are alike requited,
     God is forgotten, and the Doctor slighted.
     Robert Owen (1771–1838) British social reformer.
     Epigram

66   Every physician must be rich in knowledge, and not only of that which is

written in books; his patients should be his book, they will never mislead him.
Paracelsus (c. 1493–1541) Swiss philosopher and alchemist.
The Book of Tartaric Diseases, Ch. 13

67 The doctors were very brave about it.
Dorothy Parker (1893–1967) US writer and wit.
Journal of the American Medical Association, 194:211, 1965
Said after she had been seriously ill

68 Life in itself is short enough, but the physicians with their art, know to their amusement, how to make it still shorter.
Petrarch (1304–74) Italian poet.
Invectives, Preface, Letter to Pope Clement VI

69 After all, a doctor is just to put your mind at rest.
Petronius (fl. 1st century AD) Roman satirist.
Satyricon, 42

70 There is not a doctor who desires the health of his friends; nor a soldier who desires the peace of his country.
Philemon (c. 361 BC–c. 263 BC) Greek dramatist.
Fabulae Incertae, Fragment 46

71 A country doctor needs more brains to do his work passably than the fifty greatest industrialists in the world require.
Walter B. Pitkin
The Twilight of the American Mind

72 They are in general the most amiable companions and the best friends, as well as the most learned men I know.
Alexander Pope (1688–1744) English poet.
Letter to Ralph Allen, 13 Sept 1743

73 Who shall decide when doctors disagree.
Alexander Pope
Moral Ethics, III

74 Cur'd yesterday of my disease,
I died last night of my physician.
Matthew Prior (1664–1721) British poet.
The Remedy Worse than the Disease

75 A doctor who doesn't say too many foolish things is a patient half-cured, just as a critic is a poet who has stopped writing verse and a policeman a burglar who has retired from practice.
Marcel Proust (1871–1922) French novelist.
A la recherche du temps perdu: Le Côté de Guermantes

76 A priest sees people at their best, a lawyer at their worst, but a doctor sees
    them as they really are.
    Proverb

77 A young doctor makes a full graveyard.
    Proverb ·

78 Nature, time, and patience are the three great physicians.
    Proverb

79 While doctors consult, the patient dies.
    Proverb

80 Physicians of all men are most happy; what success soever they have, the
    world proclaimeth, and what fault they commit, the earth covereth.
    Francis Quarles (1592–1644) English poet.
    Hieroglyphics of the Life of Man

81 The best doctor in the world is the Veterinarian. He can't ask his patients
    what is the matter—he's got to just know.
    Will Rogers (1879–1935) US actor and humorist.
    The Autobiography of Will Rogers, 12

82 First they get *on*, then they get *honour*, then they get *honest*.
    Humphrey Rolleston (1862–1944) British physician.
    Confessions of an Advertising Man (David Ogilvy)
    Referring to physicians

83 The doctor occupies a seat in the front row of the stalls of the human drama,
    and is constantly watching, and even intervening in, the tragedies, comedies
    and tragi-comedies which form the raw material of the literary art.
    W. Russell, Lord Brain (1895–1966)
    The Quiet Art: a Doctor's Anthology, Foreword (R. Coope)

84 The common people say, that physicians are the class of people who kill
    other men in the most polite and courteous manner.
    John of Salisbury (c. 1115–80) English churchman, philosopher, and scholar.
    Polycraticus, Bk. II, Ch. 29

85 Doctors, priests, magistrates, and officers know men as thoroughly as if they
    had made them.
    Jean-Paul Sartre (1905–80) French philosopher, dramatist, and novelist.
    Nausea, 'Shrove Tuesday'

86 Passion, you see, can be destroyed by a doctor. It cannot be created.
    Peter Shaffer (1926–) British dramatist.
    Equus, II:35

87 The most tragic thing in the world is a sick doctor.
    George Bernard Shaw (1856–1950) Irish dramatist and critic.
    The Doctor's Dilemma, I

88 Even the fact that doctors themselves die of the very diseases they profess to
cure passes unnoticed. We do not shoot out our lips and shake our heads,
saying, 'They save others: themselves they cannot save': their reputation
stands, like an African king's palace, on a foundation of dead bodies.
George Bernard Shaw
The Doctor's Dilemma, 'Preface on Doctors'

89 Make it compulsory for a doctor using a brass plate to have inscribed on it,
in addition to the letters indicating his qualifications, the words 'Remember
that I too am mortal'.
George Bernard Shaw
The Doctor's Dilemma, 'Preface on Doctors'

90 Did you ever see a boy cultivating a moustache? Well, a middle-aged doctor
cultivating a grey head is much the same sort of spectacle.
George Bernard Shaw
The Doctor's Dilemma, 'Preface on Doctors'

91 I had rather follow you to your grave than see you owe your life to any but a
regular-bred physician.
Richard Brinsley Sheridan (1751–1816) British dramatist.
St. Patrick's Day, II:4

92 We see the physician as scientist, educator and social worker, ready to coop-
erate in teamwork, in close touch with the people he disinterestedly serves, a
friend and leader . . . the social physician protecting the people and guiding
them to a healthier and happier life.
Henry C. Sigerist (1891–1957)
Proceedings of the American Philosophical Society, 90:275, 1946

93 A young man, in whose air and countenance appeared all the uncouth grav-
ity and supercilious self-conceit of a physician piping hot from his studies.
Tobias Smollett (1721–71) English novelist and journalist.
The Adventures of Peregrine Pickle, Ch. 42

94 There are worse occupations in the world than feeling a woman's pulse.
Laurence Sterne (1713–68) Irish-born English writer and churchman.

95 The physician . . . is the flower (such as it is) of our civilization.
Robert Louis Stevenson (1850–94) Scottish writer.
Underwoods, Dedication

96 The best doctors in the world are Doctor Diet,
Doctor Quiet and Doctor Merryman.
Jonathan Swift (1667–1745) Anglo-Irish priest, satirist, and poet.

97 An unruly patient makes a harsh physician.
Publilius Syrus (fl. 1st century BC) Roman dramatist.

98   The physician is superfluous amongst the healthy.
     Tacitus (c. 55 AD–c. 120 AD) Roman historian.
     Dialogus de Oratoribus

99   This is where the strength of the physician lies, be he a quack, a homeopath
     or an allopath. He supplies the perennial demand for comfort, the craving for
     sympathy that every human sufferer feels.
     Count Leo Tolstoy (1828–1910) Russian writer.
     War and Peace, Pt. 9, Ch. 16

100 He has been a doctor a year now and has had two patients, no, three, I
     think—yes, it was three; I attended their funerals.
     Mark Twain (Samuel L. Clemens; 1835–1910) US writer.

101 The physicians are the natural attorneys of the poor and the social problems
     should largely be solved by them.
     Rudolf Virchow (1821–1902) German pathologist.
     Rudolf Virchow, 'The Doctor' (Erwin H. Ackernecht)

102 The art of medicine consists of amusing the patient while Nature cures the
     disease.
     Voltaire (François-Marie Arouet; 1694–1778) French writer and philosopher.

103 But nothing is more estimable than a physician who, having studied nature
     from his youth, knows the properties of the human body, the diseases which
     assail it, the remedies which will benefit it, exercises his art with caution,
     and pays equal attention to the rich and the poor.
     Voltaire
     A Philosophical Dictionary, 'Physicians'

104 A physician is one who pours drugs of which he knows little into a body of
     which he knows less.
     Voltaire
     Attrib.

105 I know of nothing more laughable than a doctor who does not die of old
     age.
     Voltaire
     Letter to Charles Augustin Feriol, Comte d'Argental, 6 Nov 1767

106 There are no members of society whose pursuits lead them to listen more
     frequently to what has been exquisitely termed
     The still sad music of humanity.
     Samuel Warren (1807–77)
     Diary of a Late Physician, Introduction

107 Physicians are like kings, – they brook no contradiction.
     John Webster (1580–1625) English dramatist.
     The Duchess of Malfi, V:2

108   I love doctors and hate their medicine.
       Walt Whitman (1819–92) US poet.

109   Doctors are mostly impostors. The older a doctor is and the more venerated
       he is, the more he must pretend to know everything. Of course, they grow
       worse with time. Always look for a doctor who is hated by the best doctors.
       Always seek out a bright young doctor before he comes down with
       nonsense.
       Thornton Wilder (1897–1975) US novelist and dramatist.

110   Doctors are generally dull dogs.
       John Wilson (Christopher North; 1785–1854) Scottish poet, essayist, and critic.

111   Physician art thou?–one, all eyes,
       Philosopher!–a fingering slave,
       One that would peep and botanize
       Upon his mother's grave?
       William Wordsworth (1770–1850) British poet.
       A Poet's Epitaph

DOCTORS AND PATIENTS
   See also **DOCTORS, PATIENTS.**

1   Tact is a valuable attribute in gaining practice. It consists in telling a squint-
     eyed man that he has a fine, firm chin.
     J. Chalmers Da Costa (1863–1933)
     The Trials and Triumphs of the Surgeon, Ch. 1

2   He had surrendered all reality, all dread and fear, to the doctor beside him,
     as people do.
     William Faulkner (1897–1962) US novelist.
     Light in August, Ch. 17

3   The art has three factors, the disease, the patient, and physician. The physi-
     cian is the servant of the art. The patient must co-operate with the physician
     in combating the disease.
     Hippocrates (c. 460 BC–c. 377 BC) Greek physician.
     Epidemics, I

4   Truth is the breath of life to human society. It is the food of the immortal
     spirit. Yet a single word of it may kill a man as suddenly as a drop of prussic
     acid.
     Oliver Wendell Holmes (1809–94) US writer and physician.
     Valedictory address, Harvard Commencement, 10 Mar 1858

5   I deny the lawfulness of telling a lie to a sick man for fear of alarming him.
     You have no business with consequences; you are to tell the truth. Besides,
     you are not sure what effect your telling him that he is in danger may have.
     It may bring his distemper to a crisis, and that may cure him. Of all lying, I

have the greatest abhorrence of this, because I believe it has been frequently
practised on myself.
Samuel Johnson (1709–84) English lexicographer and writer.
Life of Samuel Johnson (James Boswell)

6   There are only two classes of mankind in the world – doctors and patients.
Rudyard Kipling (1865–1936) Indian-born British writer and poet.
A Doctor's Work, address to medical students at London's Middlesex Hospital,
1 Oct 1908

7   The relationship between doctor and patient partakes of a peculiar intimacy.
It presupposes on the part of the physician not only knowledge of his fellow
men, but sympathy.... This aspect of the practice of medicine has been
designated as the art; yet I wonder whether it should not, most properly, be
called the essence.
Warfield T. Longcope (1877–1953)
Bulletin of the Johns Hopkins Hospital, 50:4, 1932

8   It is the human touch after all that counts for most in our relation with our
patients.
Robert Tuttle Morris (1857–1945)
Doctors versus Folks, Ch. 3

9   When the physician said to him, 'You have lived to be an old man,' he said,
'That is because I never employed you as my physician.'
Pausanias (fl. 479 BC) Greek traveller.
Moralia, 'Sayings of Spartans' (Plutarch)

10 The treatment of a disease may be entirely impersonal; the care of a patient
must be completely personal.
Francis Weld Peabody (1881–1927)
The Care of the Patient

11 The real work of a doctor . . . is not an affair of health centres, or public
clinics, or operating theatres, or laboratories, or hospital beds. These tech-
niques have their place in medicine, but they are not medicine. The essential
unit of medical practice is the occasion when, in the intimacy of the consult-
ing room or sick room, a person who is ill, or believes himself to be ill, seeks
the advice of a doctor whom he trusts. This is a consultation and all else in
the practice of medicine derives from it.
Sir James Calvert Spence (1892–1954)
The Purpose and Practice of Medicine, Ch. 18

12 The sick man is the garden of the physicians.
Swahili proverb

13 Who are the greatest deceivers? The doctors? And the greatest fools? The
patients?
Voltaire (François-Marie Arouet; 1694–1778) French writer and philosopher.

DRINKING
See also **ABSTINENCE**.

1 One reason I don't drink is that I want to know when I am having a good time.
Nancy Astor (1879–1964) American-born British politician.
Attrib.

2 An alcoholic has been lightly defined as a man who drinks more than his own doctor.
Alvan L. Barach (1895–)
Journal of the American Medical Association, 181:393, 1962

3 Drunkenness, the ruin of reason, the destruction of strength, premature old age, momentary death.
St. Basil the Great (c. 330–c. 379) Bishop of Caesarea in Cappadocia.
Homilies, No. XIV, Ch. 7

4 For when the wine is in, the wit is out.
Thomas Becon (1512–67) English Protestant churchman.
Catechism, 375

5 So who's in a hurry?
Robert Benchley (1889–1945) US humorist.
Attrib.
When asked whether he knew that drinking was a slow death

6 Others mocking said, These men are full of new wine.
Bible: Acts
2:13

7 Woe unto them that rise up early in the morning, that they may follow strong drink; that continue until night, till wine inflame them!
Bible: Isaiah
5:11

8 Wine is a mocker, strong drink is raging: and whosoever is deceived thereby is not wise.
Bible: Proverbs
20:1

9 Look not thou upon the wine when it is red, when it giveth his colour in the cup, when it moveth itself aright.
At the last it biteth like a serpent, and stingeth like an adder.
Bible: Proverbs
23:31–32

10   Drink no longer water, but use a little wine for thy stomach's sake and thine
     often infirmities.
     Bible: I Timothy
     5:23

11   Man, being reasonable, must get drunk;
     The best of life is but intoxication.
     George Gordon, Lord Byron (1788–1824) British poet.
     Don Juan, II

12   There's nought, no doubt, so much the spirit calms
     As rum and true religion.
     George Gordon, Lord Byron

13   Then trust me, there's nothing like drinking
     So pleasant on this side the grave;
     It keeps the unhappy from thinking,
     And makes e'en the valiant more brave.
     Charles Dibdin (1745–1814) British actor and dramatist.
     Nothing Like Grog

14   First you take a drink, then the drink takes a drink, then the drink takes
     you.
     F. Scott Fitzgerald (1896–1940) US novelist.
     Ackroyd (Jules Feiffer), '1964, May 7'

15   There are more old drunkards than old doctors.
     Benjamin Franklin (1706–90) US scientist and statesman.
     Attrib.

16   Drunkenness is never anything but a substitute for happiness. It amounts to
     buying the dream of a thing when you haven't money enough to buy the
     dreamed-of thing materially.
     André Gide (1869–1951) French novelist and critic.
     Journaux

17   A taste for drink, combined with gout,
     Had doubled him up for ever.
     W. S. Gilbert (1836–1911) British dramatist.
     The Gondoliers, I

18   He that goes to bed thirsty rises healthy.
     George Herbert (1593–1633) English poet.
     Jacula Prudentum

19   Who could have foretold, from the structure of the brain, that wine could
     derange its functions?
     Hippocrates (c. 460 BC–c. 377 BC) Greek physician.

20   If merely 'feeling good' could decide, drunkenness would be the supremely
     valid human experience.
     William James (1842–1910) US psychologist and philosopher.
     Varieties of Religious Experience

21   The sway of alcohol over mankind is unquestionably due to its power to stim-
     ulate the mystical faculties of human nature.
     William James
     The Varieties of Religious Experience, 'Mysticism'

22   A branch of the sin of drunkenness, which is the root of all sins.
     James I (1566–1625) King of England.
     A Counterblast to Tobacco

23   We drink one another's health and spoil our own.
     Jerome K. Jerome (1859–1927) British humorous writer.
     Idle Thoughts of an Idle Fellow, 'On Eating and Drinking'

24   If we heard it said of Orientals that they habitually drank a liquor which
     went to their heads, deprived them of reason and made them vomit, we
     should say: 'How very barbarous!'
     Jean de La Bruyère (1645–96) French writer and moralist.
     Caractères

25   My experience through life has convinced me that, while moderation and
     temperance in all things are commendable and beneficial, abstinence from
     spirituous liquors is the best safeguard of morals and health.
     Robert E. Lee (1807–70) US general.
     Letter, 9 Dec 1869

26   Long quaffing maketh a short lyfe.
     John Lyly (1554–1606) English dramatist and novelist.
     Euphues

27   The tranquilizer of greatest value since the early history of man, and which
     may never become outdated, is alcohol, when administered in moderation. It
     possesses the distinct advantage of being especially pleasant to the taste buds.
     Nathan Masor (1913–   )
     Attrib.

28   Candy
     Is dandy
     But liquor
     Is quicker.
     Ogden Nash (1902–71) US poet.
     Hard Lines, 'Reflection on Ice-Breaking'

29   Two great European narcotics, alcohol and Christianity.
     Friedrich Nietzsche (1844–1900) German philosopher and poet.
     The Twilight of the Idols, 'Things the Germans Lack'

30 Wine is the most healthful and most hygienic of beverages.
Louis Pasteur (1822–95) French scientist.
Etudes sur le vin, Pt. I, Ch. 2

31 Drunkenness . . . spoils health, dismounts the mind, and unmans men.
William Penn (1644–1718) English founder of Pennsylvania.
Fruits of Solitude, Maxim 72

32 There are more old drunkards than old doctors.
Proverb

33 The brewery is the best drugstore.
Proverb

34 Drunkenness is temporary suicide: the happiness that it brings is merely negative, a momentary cessation of unhappiness.
Bertrand Russell (1872–1970) British philosopher.

35 Drink a glass of wine after your soup, and you steal a ruble from the doctor.
Russian proverb

36 'Tis not the drinking that is to be blamed, but the excess.
John Selden (1584–1654) English historian.
Table Talk

37 Drunkenness is simply voluntary insanity.
Seneca (c. 4 BC–AD 65) Roman writer.
Epistulae ad Lucilium, LXXXIII

38 It provokes the desire, but it takes away the performance. Therefore much drink may be said to be an equivocator with lechery.
William Shakespeare (1564–1616) English dramatist and poet.
Macbeth, II:3

39 MACDUFF. What three things does drink especially provoke?
PORTER. Marry, sir, nose-painting, sleep, and urine.
William Shakespeare
Macbeth, II:3

40 Well, then, my stomach must just digest in its waistcoat.
Richard Brinsley Sheridan (1751–1816) British dramatist.
The Fine Art of Political Wit (L. Harris)
On being warned that his drinking would destroy the coat of his stomach

41 There are two things that will be believed of any man whatsoever, and one of them is that he has taken to drink.
Booth Tarkington (1869–1946) US novelist.
Penrod, Ch. 10

42 An alcoholic is someone you don't like who drinks as much as you do.
Dylan Thomas (1914–53) Welsh poet.
Dictionary of 20th Century Quotations (Nigel Rees)

43 Eat everything, drink everything and don't worry about anything. Its always
    nice to have a shot just before breakfast.
    Mrs. Galsomina Del Vecchio
    Bartlett's Unfamiliar Quotations (Leonard Louis Levinson)
    Said at the age of 108

DRUGS
See also **NARCOTICS.**

1   A drug is that substance which, when injected into a rat, will produce a sci-
    entific report.
    Anonymous

2   Hark! The herald angels sing
    Beecham's pills are just the thing.
    Peace on earth and mercy mild;
    Two for man and one for child.
    Anonymous

3   Modern therapy, particularly of malignancy, makes good use of the Borgia ef-
    fect—two poisons are more efficacious than one.
    Anonymous

4   APOTHECARY, n. The physician's accomplice, undertaker's benefactor and
    grave worm's provider.
    Ambrose Bierce (1842–c. 1914) US writer and journalist.
    The Devil's Dictionary

5   Better to hunt in fields for health unbought,
    Than fee the doctor for a nauseous draught.
    John Dryden (1631–1700) English poet and dramatist.
    To Sir G. Kneller

6   The poisons are our principal medicines, which kill the disease and save the
    life.
    Ralph Waldo Emerson (1803–82) US poet and essayist.
    The Conduct of Life, Ch. 7

7   A man who cannot work without his hypodermic needle is a poor doctor.
    The amount of narcotic you use is inversely proportional to your skill.
    Martin H. Fischer (1879–1962)
    Fischerisms (Howard Fabing and Ray Marr)

8   Half the modern drugs could well be thrown out the window, except that the
    birds might eat them.
    Martin H. Fischer
    Fischerisms (Howard Fabing and Ray Marr)

9 He's the best physician that knows the worthlessness of the most medicines.
Benjamin Franklin (1706–90) US scientist and statesman.
Poor Richard's Almanac

10 Keep a watch also on the faults of the patients, which often make them lie about the taking of things prescribed.
Hippocrates (c. 460 BC–c. 377 BC) Greek physician.
Decorum, 14

11 A miracle drug is any drug that will do what the label says it will do.
Eric Hodgins (1899–1971) US writer and editor.
Episode

12 No families take so little medicine as those of doctors, except those of apothecaries.
Oliver Wendell Holmes (1809–94) US writer and physician.
Medical Essays, 'Currents and Counter-Currents in Medical Science'

13 A hundred doses of happiness are not enough: send to the drug-store for another bottle—and, when that is finished, for another. . . . There can be no doubt that, if tranquillizers could be bought as easily and cheaply as aspirin they would be consumed, not by the billions, as they are at present, but by the scores and hundreds of billions. And a good, cheap stimulant would be almost as popular.
Aldous Huxley (1894–1964) British writer.
Brave New World Revisited, Ch. 8

14 One of the most successful physicians I have ever known, has assured me, that he used more bread pills, drops of colored water, and powders of hickory ashes, than of all other medicines put together. It was certainly a pious fraud.
Thomas Jefferson (1743–1826) US statesman.
Letter to Dr. Caspar Wistar, 21 June 1807

15 The patient, treated on the fashionable theory, sometimes gets well in spite of the medicine. The medicine therefore restored him, and the young doctor receives new courage to proceed in his bold experiments on the lives of his fellow creatures.
Thomas Jefferson
Letter to Dr. Caspar Wistar, 21 June 1807

16 Poisons and medicine are oftentimes the same substance given with different intents.
Peter Mere Latham (1789–1875) US poet and essayist.
General Remarks on the Practice of Medicine, Ch. 7

17 What is dangerous about the tranquilizers is that whatever peace of mind they bring is a packaged peace of mind. Where you buy a pill and buy peace with it, you get conditioned to cheap solutions instead of deep ones.
Max Lerner (1902–) Russian-born US teacher, editor, and journalist.
The Unfinished Country, 'The Assault on the Mind'

18   He felt about books as doctors feel about medicines, or managers about plays—
     cynical but hopeful.
     Dame Rose Macaulay (1881–1958) British writer.
     Crewe Train, Ch. 8, Pt. 2

19   I will lift up mine eyes unto the pills. Almost everyone takes them, from the
     humble aspirin to the multi-coloured, king-sized three deckers, which put you
     to sleep, wake you up, stimulate and soothe you all in one. It is an age of
     pills.
     Malcolm Muggeridge (1903–   ) British writer and editor.
     The New Statesman, 3 Aug 1962

20   Medicines are only fit for old people.
     Napoleon I (Napoleon Bonaparte; 1769–1821) French Emperor.
     Napoleon in Exile (Barry O'Meara)

21   One of the first duties of the physician is to educate the masses not to take
     medicine.
     Sir William Osler (1849–1919) Canadian physician.
     Sir William Osler: Aphorisms, Ch. 3 (William B. Bean)

22   Imperative drugging – the ordering of medicine in any and every malady – is
     no longer regarded as the chief function of the doctor.
     Sir William Osler
     Aequanimitas, with Other Addresses, 'Medicine in the Nineteenth Century'

23   Many medicines, few cures.
     Proverb

24   The best practitioners give to their patients the least medicine.
     Frederick Saunders (1807–1902)

25   It is medicine not scenery, for which a sick man must go searching.
     Seneca (4 BC–65 AD) Roman writer and statesman.
     Epistulae ad Lucilium, CIV

26   The medicine increases the disease.
     Virgil (Publius Vergilius Maro; 70 BC–19 BC) Roman poet.
     Aeneid, Bk. XII

27   I owe my reputation to the fact that I use digitalis in doses the text books say
     are dangerous and in cases that the text books say are unsuitable.
     Karel Frederik Wenckebach (1864–1940)
     Lancet, 2:633, 1937

DYING
     See **DEATH.**

E

EATING
See also **HEALTHY EATING.**

1   EAT, v.i. To perform successively (and successfully) the functions of mastication, humectation, and deglutition.
Ambrose Bierce (1842–c. 1914) US writer and journalist.
The Devil's Dictionary

EDUCATION
See **MEDICAL STUDENTS.**

ENDURANCE

1   What can't be cured, must be endured.
Proverb

2   O you who have borne even heavier things, God will grant an end to these too.
Virgil (Publius Vergilius Maro; 70 BC–19 BC) Roman poet.
Aeneid, Bk. I

ENVIRONMENT

1   The first Care in building of Cities, is to make them airy and well perflated; infectious Distempers must necessarily be propagated amongst Mankind living close together.
John Arbuthnot 1667–1735) Scottish physician and satirist.
An Essay Concerning the Effects of Air on Human Bodies

2   As cruel a weapon as the cave man's club, the chemical barrage has been hurled against the fabric of life.
Rachel Carson (1907–64) US marine biologist and writer.
The Silent Spring

3   It can be said that each civilization has a pattern of disease peculiar to it. The pattern of disease is an expression of the response of man to his total environment (physical, biological, and social); this response is, therefore, determined by anything that affects man himself or his environment.
René J. Dubos (1901–   )
Industrial Medicine and Surgery, 30:369, 1961

4   I say that it touches a man that his blood is sea water and his tears are salt, that the seed of his loins is scarcely different from the same cells in a sea-weed, and that of stuff like his bones are coral made. I say that a physical and biologic law lies down with him, and wakes when a child stirs in the womb, and that the sap in a tree, uprushing in the spring, and the smell of the loam, where the darkness, and the path of the sun in the heaven, these are facts of first importance to his mental conclusions, and that a man who goes in no consciousness of them is a drifter and a dreamer, without a home or any contact with reality.
    Donald Culross Peattie (1898–1964)
    An Almanac for Moderns, 'April First'

5   It is obvious that the best qualities in man must atrophy in a standing-room-only environment.
    Stewart L. Udall (1920– .) US politician.
    The Quiet Crisis, 13

EPIDEMICS

1   For I will pass through the land of Egypt this night, and will smite all the firstborn in the land of Egypt, both man and beast; and against all the gods of Egypt I will execute judgment: I am the Lord.
    Bible: Exodus
    12:12

2   Epidemics have often been more influential than statesmen and soldiers in shaping the course of political history, and diseases may also color the moods of civilizations.
    René and Jean Dubos (1901– ; 1918–)
    The White Plague, Ch. 5

3   Some people are so sensitive they feel snubbed if an epidemic overlooks them.
    Frank (Kin) Hubbard (1868–1930) US humorist and journalist.
    Abe Martin's Broadcast

4   In scarcely any house did only one die, but all together, man and wife with their children and household, traversed the same road, the road of death . . . I leave the parchment for the work to be continued in case in the future any human survivor should remain, or someone of the race of Adam should be able to escape this plague and continue what I have begun.
    John of Clyn (fl. 14th century) Irish friar.
    Annals of Ireland
    Recording the effects of the Black Death in Kilkenny

5   Thence I walked to the Tower; but Lord! how empty the streets are and how melancholy, so many poor sick people in the streets full of sores . . . in West-

minster, there is never a physician and but one apothecary left, all being dead.
Samuel Pepys (1633–1703) English diarist.
Diary, 16 Sept 1665
Written during the Great Plague – the last major outbreak of bubonic plague in England, and the worst since the Black Death of 1348

ETHICS
See **MEDICAL ETHICS.**

EUTHANASIA

1   Euthanasia is a long, smooth-sounding word, and it conceals its danger as long, smooth words do, but the danger is there, nevertheless.
Pearl Buck (1892–1973) US novelist.
The Child Who Never Grew, Ch. 2

2   Thou shalt not kill; but needst not strive
Officiously to keep alive.
Arthur Hugh Clough (1819–61) British poet.
The Latest Decalogue, 11

3   To save a man's life against his will is the same as killing him.
Horace (Quintus Horatius Flaccus; 65 BC–8 BC) Roman poet.
Ars Poetica

4   It is the duty of a doctor to prolong life. It is not his duty to prolong the act of dying.
Lord Thomas Horder (1871–1955)
Speech in the House of Lords, Dec 1936

5   To kill a human being is, after all, the least injury you can do him.
Henry James (1843–1916) US novelist.
My Friend Bingham

6   Death is a punishment to some, to some a gift, and to many a favour.
Seneca (c. 4 BC–AD 65) Roman writer.
Hercules Oetaeus

7   Death is not the greatest of ills, it is worse to want to die, and not to be able to.
Sophocles (c. 496 BC–406 BC) Greek dramatist.
Electra

EVOLUTION

1   Descended from the apes? My dear, we will hope it is not true. But if it is, let us pray that it may not become generally known.
Anonymous
Man's Most Dangerous Myth, The Fallacy of Race (F. Ashley Montagu)
Remark by the wife of a canon of Worcester Cathedral

2   Progress is
The law of life, man is not man as yet.
Robert Browning (1812–89) British poet.
Paracelsus, 5

3   A hen is only an egg's way of making another egg.
Samuel Butler (1835–1902) British writer.
Life and Habit, VIII

4   Some call it Evolution
And others call it God.
William H. Carruth (1859–1924)
Each in His Own Tongue

5   I confess freely to you I could never look long upon a Monkey, without very Mortifying Reflections.
William Congreve (1670–1729) English Restoration dramatist.
Letter to John Dennis, 10 July 1695

6   We must, however, acknowledge, as it seems to me, that man with all his noble qualities, still bears in his bodily frame the indelible stamp of his lowly origin.
Charles Darwin (1809–82) British life scientist.
Descent of Man, Ch. 21
Closing words

7   The expression often used by Mr. Herbert Spencer of the Survival of the Fittest is more accurate, and is sometimes equally convenient.
Charles Darwin
Origin of Species, Ch. 3

8   We will now discuss in a little more detail the struggle for existence.
Charles Darwin
Origin of Species, Ch. 3

9   I have called this principle, by which each slight variation, if useful, is preserved, by the term of Natural Selection.
Charles Darwin
Origin of Species, Ch. 3

10   The question is this: Is man an ape or an angel? I, my lord, am on the side
     of the angels.
     Benjamin Disraeli (1804–81) British statesman.
     Speech, 25 Nov 1864

11   How like us is that ugly brute, the ape!
     Ennius (239 BC–169 BC) Roman poet.
     On the Nature of the Gods, I (Cicero)

12   I am, in point of fact, a particularly haughty and exclusive person, of pre-Ad-
     amite ancestral descent. You will understand this when I tell you that I can
     trace my ancestry back to a protoplasmal primordic atomic globule.
     William S. Gilbert (1836–1911) British dramatist and comic writer.
     The Mikado, I

13   Philip is a living example of natural selection. He was as fitted to survive in
     this modern world as a tapeworm in an intestine.
     William Golding (1911–   ) British novelist.
     Free Fall, Ch. 2

14   I am quite sure that our views on evolution would be very different had bi-
     ologists studied genetics and natural selection before and not after most of
     them were convinced that evolution had occurred.
     J. B. S. Haldane (1892–1964) British geneticist.

15   Everything from an egg.
     William Harvey (1578–1657) English physician.
     De Generatione Animalium, Frontispiece

16   The probable fact is that we are descended not only from monkeys but from
     monks.
     Elbert G. Hubbard (1856–1915) US writer and editor.
     A Thousand and One Epigrams

17   I asserted – and I repeat – that a man has no reason to be ashamed of hav-
     ing an ape for his grandfather. If there were an ancestor whom I should feel
     shame in recalling it would rather be a *man* – a man of restless and versatile
     intellect – who, not content with an equivocal success in his own sphere of
     activity, plunges into scientific questions with which he has no real acquain-
     tance, only to obscure them by an aimless rhetoric, and distract the attention
     of his hearers from the real point at issue by eloquent digressions and skilled
     appeals to religious prejudice.
     T. H. Huxley (1825–95) British biologist.
     Speech, 30 June 1860
     Replying to Bishop Wilberforce. After hearing Wilberforce's speech Huxley is
     said to have remarked, 'The Lord has delivered him into my hands!'

18   Evolution is far more important than living.
     Ernst Jünger
     The Rebel, Ch. 3 (Albert Camus)

19 We are very slightly changed
From the semi-apes who ranged
India's prehistoric clay.
Rudyard Kipling (1865–1936) Indian-born British writer.
General Summary

20 Man appears to be the missing link between anthropoid apes and human beings.
Konrad Lorenz (1903–) Austrian zoologist and pioneer of ethology.
The New York Times Magazine, 11 Apr 1965 (John Pfeiffer)

21 Species do not evolve toward perfection, but quite the contrary. The weak, in fact, always prevail over the strong, not only because they are in the majority, but also because they are the more crafty.
Friedrich Nietzsche (1844–1900) German philosopher.
The Twilight of the Idols

22 An ape is ne'er so like an ape
As when he wears a doctor's cape.
Proverb

23 The tide of evolution carries everything before it, thoughts no less than bodies, and persons no less than nations.
George Santayana (1863–1952) Spanish-born US philosopher, poet, and critic.
Little Essays, 44

24 Survival of the fittest.
Herbert Spencer (1820–1903) British philosopher.
Principles of Biology, Pt. III, Ch. 12

25 We have been God-like in our planned breeding of our domesticated plants and animals, but we have been rabbit-like in our unplanned breeding of ourselves.
Arnold Toynbee (1889–1975) British historian.
National Observer, 10 June 1963

26 And, in conclusion, I would like to ask the gentleman . . . whether the ape from which he is descended was on his grandmother's or his grandfather's side of the family.
Samuel Wilberforce (1805–73) British churchman.
In a debate on Darwin's theory at the meeting of the British Association for the Advancement of Science in Oxford, 30 June 1860

EXERCISE
See also **HEALTHY LIVING.**

1 I have two doctors—my left leg and my right.
Anonymous

2   It is a fact that not once in all my life have I gone out for a walk. I have
    been taken out for walks; but that is another matter.
    Max Beerbohm (1872–1956) British writer.
    Going Out of a Walk

3   I get my exercise acting as a pallbearer to my friends who exercise.
    Chauncey Depew (1834–1928) US politician.
    Attrib.

4   Those who think they have not time for bodily exercise will sooner or later
    have to find time for illness.
    Edward Stanley, Earl of Derby (1826–93) British statesman.
    The Conduct of Life, address at Liverpool College, 20 Dec 1873

5   Exercise is bunk. If you are healthy, you don't need it: if you are sick, you
    shouldn't take it.
    Henry Ford (1863–1947) US car manufacturor.
    Attrib.

6   Fat people who want to reduce should take their exercise on an empty stom-
    ach and sit down to their food out of breath . . . . Thin people who want to
    get fat should do exactly the opposite and never take exercise on an empty
    stomach.
    Hippocrates (c. 460 BC–c. 377 BC) Greek physician.
    A Regimen for Health, IV

7   The Greeks understood that mind and body must develop in harmonious pro-
    portions to produce a creative intelligence. And so did the most brilliant in-
    telligence of our earliest days–Thomas Jefferson–when he said, not less than
    two hours a day should be devoted to exercise.
    If the man who wrote the Declaration of Independence, was Secretary of
    State, and twice President, could give it two hours, our children can give it
    ten or fifteen minutes.
    John F. Kennedy (1917–1963) US statesman.
    Address to the National Football Foundation, 5 Dec 1961

8   The only exercise I get is when I take the studs out of one shirt and put
    them in another.
    Ring Lardner Jnr. (1885–1933) US humorist.
    Bartlett's Unfamiliar Quotations (Leonard Louis Levinson)

EXPERIENCE

1   Inexperience is what makes a young man do what an older man says is
    impossible.
    Herbert V. Prochnow (1897–   ) US writer.
    Saturday Evening Post, 4 Dec 1948

EYES

1   'Yes I have a pair of eyes,' replied Sam, 'and that's just it. If they was a pair
    o' patent double million magnifyin' gas microscopes of hextra power, p'raps I
    might be able to see through a flight o' stairs and a deal door; but bein' only
    eyes, you see, my vision's limited.'
    Charles Dickens (1812–70) British novelist.
    The Pickwick Papers

2   That youthful sparkle in his eyes is caused by his contact lenses, which he
    keeps highly polished.
    Sheilah Graham
    The Times, 22 Aug 1981
    Referring to Ronald Reagan

3   Who formed the curious texture of the eye,
    And cloath'd it with the various tunicles,
    And texture exquisite; with chrystal juice
    Supply'd it, to transmit the rays of light?
    Henry Needler (1685–1760)
    A Poem to Prove the Certainty of a God

F

FADS

1 Medicine is like a woman who changes with the fashions.
   August Bier (1861–1949)
   Aphorism

2 Alarmed successively by every fashionable medical terror of the day, she dosed
   her children with every specific which was publicly advertised or privately
   recommended. No creatures of their age had taken such quantities of Ching's
   lozenges, Godbold's elixir, or Dixon's anti-bilious pills. The consequence was,
   that the dangers, which had at first been imaginary, became real: these little
   victims of domestic medicine never had a day's health: they looked, and
   were, more dead than alive.
   Maria Edgeworth (1767–1849) British novelist.
   Patronage

3 The doctors are always changing their opinions. They always have some new
   fad.
   David Lloyd George (1863–1945) British Liberal statesman.
   War Diary, Ch. 36 (Lord Riddell)
   After being informed that a well-known surgeon recommended that people
   sleep on their stomachs

4 I haven't the slightest idea where fashions in pathology are born. . . .
   Possibly some of my older readers dimly recollect the days when modish
   scientists declared that the only dependable method of relieving a toothache
   was a clean, conclusive appendectomy. Then the whistle blew for the quarter,
   the two teams changed goals, and it developed that if you had a pain in your
   side it was high time your teeth came out . . . . Only one point is clear: it's
   better to be dead, or even perfectly well, than to suffer from the wrong affliction. The man who owns up to affliction. The man who owns up to arthritis
   in a beriberi year is as lonely as a woman in a last month's dress.
   Ogden Nash (1902–71) US poet.
   Saturday Evening Post, 14 Oct 1933

FAITH

1 There was a faith-healer of Deal,
   Who said, 'Although pain isn't real,
   If I sit on a pin
   And it punctures my skin,

I dislike what I fancy I feel.'
Anonymous

2 The prayer of faith shall save the sick.
Bible: James
5:15

3 Optimism: A kind of heart stimulant – the digitalis of failure.
Elbert G. Hubbard (1856–1915)
The Roycroft Dictionary

4 Nothing in life is more wonderful than faith–the one great moving force
which we can neither weigh in the balance nor test in the crucible.
Sir William Osler (1849–1919) Canadian physician.
British Medical Journal, 1:1470, 1910

5 Life is doubt, and faith without doubt is nothing but death.
Miguel de Unamuno y Jugo (1864–1936) Spanish writer and philosopher.
Poesías

6 There can be no scientific dispute with respect to faith, for science and faith
exclude one another.
Rudolf Virchow (1821–1902) German pathologist.
Disease, Life, and Man, 'On Man'

FAMILY

1 He that hath wife and children hath given hostages to fortune; for they are
impediments to great enterprises, either of virtue or mischief.
Sir Francis Bacon (1561–1626) English philosopher, lawyer, and politician.
Essays, 'Of Marriage and Single Life'

2 Far from being the basis of the good society, the family, with its narrow pri-
vacy and tawdry secrets, is the source of all our discontents.
Edmund Leach (1910–) British social anthropologist.
In the BBC Reith Lectures for 1967. Lecture reprinted in *The Listener*

3 The sink is the great symbol of the bloodiness of family life. All life is bad,
but family life is worse.
Julian Mitchell (1935–) British writer.
As Far as You Can Go, Pt. I, Ch. 1

4 That dear octopus from whose tentacles we never quite escape, nor in our in-
nermost hearts never quite wish to.
Dodie Smith (1896–) British dramatist and novelist.
Dear Octopus

5   All happy families resemble one another, each unhappy family is unhappy in
    its own way.
    Leo Tolstoy (1828–1910) Russian writer.
    Anna Karenina, Pt. I, Ch. 1

FEES
    See **MEDICAL FEES.**

FERTILITY

1   The moon is nothing
    But a circumambulating aphrodisiac
    Divinely subsidized to provoke the world
    Into a rising birth-rate.
    Christopher Fry (1907–   ) British dramatist.
    The Lady's Not for Burning

2   The management of fertility is one of the most important functions of
    adulthood.
    Germaine Greer (1939–   ) Australian-born British writer and feminist.

3   Common morality now treats childbearing as an aberration. There are practi-
    cally no good reasons left for exercising one's fertility.
    Germaine Greer

4   Why should human females become sterile in the forties, while female croco-
    diles continue to lay eggs into their third century?
    Aldous Huxley (1894–1964) British writer.
    After Many a Summer, I, Ch. 5

FEVER

1   Once Antigonis was told his son, Demetrius, was ill, and went to see him.
    At the door he met some young beauty. Going in, he sat down by the bed
    and took his pulse. 'The fever,' said Demetrius, 'has just left me.' 'Oh, yes,'
    replied the father, 'I met it going out at the door.'
    Plutarch (c. 46 AD– c. 120 AD) Greek biographer and essayist.
    Bartlett's Unfamiliar Quotations (Leonard Louis Levinson)

FIRST˙AID

1   I've already had medical attention, a dog licked me when I was on the
    ground.
    Neil Simon (1927–   ) US playwright.
    Only When I Laugh (screenplay)

FOOD
See EATING, HEALTHY EATING.

G

GENERAL PRACTITIONERS
See also **ANATOMY, CONSULTANTS, DOCTORS, SURGEONS.**

1   'I haven't got time to be sick!' he said. 'People need me.' For he was a country doctor, and he did not know what it was to spare himself.
Don Marquis (1878–1937) US journalist and writer.
Country Doctor

2   A general practitioner can no more become a specialist than an old shoe can become a dancing slipper. Both have developed habits which are immutable.
Frank Kittredge Paddock (1841–1901)
Aphorism

3   A country doctor needs more brains to do his work passably than the fifty greatest industrialists in the world require.
Walter B. Pitkin (1878–1953)
The Twilight of the American Mind, Ch. 10

GERMS

1   In the Nineteenth Century men lost their fear of God and acquired a fear of microbes.
Anonymous

2   The Microbe is so very small
You cannot make him out at all,
But many sanguine people hope
To see him through a microscope.
His jointed tongue that lies beneath
A hundred curious rows of teeth;
His seven tufted tails with lots
Of lovely pink and purple spots,
On each of which a pattern stands,
Composed of forty separate bands;
His eyebrows of a tender green;
But Scientists, who ought to know,
Assure us that they must be so . . . .
Oh! let us never, never doubt
What nobody is sure about!
Hilaire Belloc (1870–1953) French-born British poet, essayist and historian.
Cautionary Verses, 'The Microbe'

3   There are more microbes *per person* than the entire population of the world.

Imagine that. Per person. This means that if the time scale is diminished in proportion to that of space it would be quite possible for the whole story of Greece and Rome to be played out between farts.
Alan Bennett (1934–   ) British dramatist and actor.
The Old Country, II

4   Oh, powerful bacillus,
With wonder how you fill us,
Every day!
While medical detectives,
With powerful objectives,
Watch your play.
William T. Helmuth (1833–1902)
Ode to the Bacillus

GOUT

1   'Pray, Mr. Abernethy, what is a cure for gout?' was the question of an indolent and luxurious citizen. 'Live upon sixpence a day – and earn it,' was the cogent reply.
John Abernethy (1764–1831) English surgeon.
Medical Portrait Gallery, Vol. II (Thomas J. Pettigrew)

2   Screw up the vise as tightly as possible—you have rheumatism; give it another turn, and that is gout.
Anonymous

3   Punch cures the gout, the colic, and the 'tsick
And is by all agreed the very best of physic.
Anonymous
English rhyme (18th Century)

4   GOUT, n. A physician's name for the rheumatism of a rich patient.
Ambrose Bierce (1842–c. 1914) US writer and journalist.
The Devil's Dictionary

5   There is, however, a pathological condition which occurs so often, in such extreme forms, and in men of such pre-eminent intellectual ability, that it is impossible not to regard it as having a real association with such ability. I refer to gout.
Havelock Ellis (1859–1939) British psychologist.
A Study of British Genius, Ch. 8

6   To think that a bottle of wine or a truffled pâté, or even a glass of beer, instead of being absorbed and eliminated by the system in the usual manner, should mine its way through the thighs, knees, calves, ankles, and instep, to

explode at last in a fiery volcano in one's great toe, seems a mirth-provoking
phenomenon to all but him who is immediately concerned.
George Herman Ellwanger (fl. 1897)
Meditations on Gout, 'The Malady'

7   'In our case,' says the Frenchman, addressing the Englishman, 'we have 'goût'
    for the taste; in your case, you have 'gout' for the result!'
    George Herman Ellwanger
    Meditations on Gout, 'The Theory'

8   Time had robbed her of her personal charms, and that scourge of the human
    race, the gout, was racking her bones and sinews.
    Hannah Farnham Lee (1780–1865)
    The Huguenots in France and America
    Referring to Catherine de Medici

9   It is with jealousy as with the gout. When such distempers are in the blood,
    there is never any security against their breaking out; and that often on the
    slightest occasions, and when least suspected.
    Henry Fielding (1707–54) English writer.
    Tom Jones, Bk. II, Ch. 3

10 If gentlemen love the pleasant titillation of the gout, it is all one to the
    Town Pump.
    Nathaniel Hawthorne (1804–64) US writer.
    The Town Pump

11 For that old enemy the gout
    Had taken him in toe!
    Thomas Hood (1799–1845) British poet and humorist.
    Lieutenant Luff

12 Gout is to the arteries what rheumatism is to the heart.
    Henri Huchard (1844–1910)
    Lancet, 1:164, 1967 (D. Evan Bedford)

13 My corns ache, I get gouty, and my prejudices swell like varicose veins.
    James Gibbons Huneker (1860–1921)
    Old Fogy, Ch. 1

14 Drink wine, and have the gout; drink no wine, and have the gout too.
    Proverb

15 Oh! when I have the gout, I feel as if I was walking on my eyeballs.
    Sydney Smith (1771–1845) English churchman, essayist, and wit.
    A Memoir of the Rev. Sydney Smith, Ch. 11 (Lady Holland)

16 The old saw is that 'if you drink wine you have the gout, and if you do not
    drink wine the gout will have you.'
    Thomas Sydenham (1624–89)
    Works, 'A Treatise on Gout and Dropsy'

H

HANGOVERS

1 His mouth has been used as a latrine by some small animal of the night.
Kingsley Amis (1922–) British novelist.
Lucky Jim
Describing a hangover

HAY FEVER
See also **ALLERGIES.**

1 Hay fever is the real Flower Power.
Leonard Louis Levinson
Bartlett's Unfamiliar Quotations (Leonard Louis Levinson)

HEALING
See also **CURES, DIAGNOSIS, REMEDIES, TREATMENT.**

1 Visitors' footfalls are like medicine; they heal the sick.
Bantu (Chuana) proverb

2 Time is a physician that heals every grief.
Diphilius (4th century BC)

3 Healing is a matter of time, but it is sometimes also a matter of opportunity.
Hippocrates (c. 460 BC–c. 377 BC) Greek physician.
Precepts, I

4 Common sense is in medicine the master workman.
Peter Mere Latham (1789–1875) US poet and essayist.
General Remarks on the Practice of Medicine, Ch. 5

5 Wounds heal and become scars. But scars grow with us.
Stanislaw Lec (1909–) Polish poet.
Unkempt Thoughts

6 Time heals what reason cannot.
Seneca (c. 4 BC–65 AD) Roman writer and statesman.
Agamemnon, 130

HEALTH
See also **HEALTH CARE, HEALTHY EATING, HEALTHY LIVING.**

1   Health is the first of all liberties, and happiness gives us the energy which is
    the basis of health.
    Henri Amiel (1821–81) Swiss philosopher and writer.
    Journal intime, 3 Apr 1865

2   In sickness, respect health principally; and in health, action. For those that
    put their bodies to endure in health, may in most sicknesses, which are not
    very sharp, be cured only with diet and tendering.
    Sir Francis Bacon (1561–1626) English philosopher, lawyer, and politician.
    Essays, 'Of Regiment of Health'

3   Health indeed is a precious thing, to recover and preserve which, we undergo
    any misery, drink bitter potions, freely give our goods: restore a man to his
    health, his purse lies open to thee.
    Robert Burton (1577–1640) English scholar and explorer.
    The Anatomy of Melancholy, Pt. III, Sect. 1

4   The health of people is really the foundation upon which all their happiness
    and all their power as a State depend.
    Benjamin Disraeli, Lord Beaconsfield (1804–81) British statesman.
    Speech, 23 June 1877

5   We're all of us ill in one way or another:
    We call it health when we find no symptom
    Of illness. Health is a relative term.
    T. S. Eliot (1888–1965) US-born British poet and dramatist.
    The Family Reunion, I:3

6   Give me health and a day, and I will make the pomp of emperors ridiculous.
    Ralph Waldo Emerson (1803–82) US poet and essayist.
    Nature, Addresses and Lectures, 'Beauty'

7   HEALTHY: Too much health, the cause of illness.
    Gustave Flaubert (1821–80) French novelist.
    Dictionary of Accepted Ideas

8   A wise man ought to realize that health is his most valuable possession.
    Hippocrates (c. 460 BC–c. 377 BC) Greek physician.
    A Regimen for Health, 9

9   If I had my way I'd make health catching instead of disease.
    Robert G. Ingersoll (1833–99) US lawyer and agnostic.

10 O health! health! the blessing of the rich! the riches of the poor! who can
    buy thee at too deare a rate, since there is no enjoying this world, without
    thee?
    Ben Jonson (1573–1637) English dramatist.
    Volpone, II:2

11 Your prayer must be for a sound mind in a sound body.
Juvenal (Decimus Junius Juvenalis; c. 60 AD–130 AD) Roman satirist.
Satires, X

12 Life is not living, but living in health.
Martial (c. 40 AD–c. 104 AD) Roman poet.
Epigrams, VI

13 Good health is an essential to happiness, and happiness is an essential to good citizenship.
Charles H. Mayo (1865–1939) US physician.
Journal of the American Dental Association, 6:505, 1919

14 Health is a precious thing, and the only one, in truth, which deserves that we employ in its pursuit not only time, sweat, trouble, and worldly goods, but even life; inasmuch as without it life comes to be painful and oppressive to us . . . As far as I am concerned, no road that would lead us to health is either arduous or expensive.
Michel de Montaigne (1533–92) French essayist and moralist.
Essays, II

15 A good wife and health are a man's best wealth.
Proverb

16 Without health life is not life; it is unlivable. . . . Without health, life spells but languor and an image of death.
François Rabelais (c. 1483–1553) French humanist and satirist.
Pantagruel, Bk. IV, Prologue

17 To preserve one's health by too strict a regime is in itself a tedious malady.
Duc François de La Rochefoucauld (1613–80) French writer.
Maxims, 623

18 All health is better than wealth.
Sir Walter Scott (1771–1832) Scottish novelist.
Familiar Letters, Letter to C. Carpenter, 4 Aug 1812

19 Health is beauty, and the most perfect health is the most perfect beauty.
William Shenstone (1714–63) English poet.
Essays on Men and Manners, 'On Taste'

20 The preservation of health is a duty. Few seem conscious that there is such a thing as physical morality.
Herbert Spencer (1820–1903) British philosopher.

21 'Tis healthy to be sick sometimes.
Henry David Thoreau (1817–62) US writer.

22 Look to your health: and if you have it, praise God, and value it next to a

good conscience; for health is the second blessing that we mortals are capable of; a blessing that money cannot buy.
Izaak Walton (1593–1683) English writer.
The Compleat Angler, Pt. I, Ch. 21

23   Gold that buys health can never be ill spent.
John Webster and Thomas Dekker (c. 1580–c. 1625; c. 1572–c. 1632) English dramatists.
Westward Ho!, V

24   Talk health. The dreary, never-ending tale
Our mortal maladies is worn and stale;
You cannot charm or interest or please
By harping on that minor chord, disease.
Say you are well, or all is well with you,
And God shall hear your words and make them true.
Ella Wheeler Wilcox (1850–1919) US poet.
Speech

HEALTH CARE

1   Effective health care depends on self-care; this fact is currently heralded as if it were a discovery . . . The medicalization of early diagnosis not only hampers and discourages preventative health-care but it also trains the patient-to-be to function in the meantime as an acolyte to his doctor. He learns to depend on the physician in sickness and in health. He turns into a life-long patient.
Ivan Illich (1926–) Austrian sociologist.
Medical Nemesis

2   No costs have increased more rapidly in the last decade than the cost of medical care. And no group of Americans has felt the impact of these sky-rocketing costs more than our older citizens.
John F. Kennedy (1917–1963) US statesman.
Address on the 25th Anniversary of the Social Security Act, 14 Aug 1960

3   Ready money is ready medicine.
Latin Proverb

4   The problem of economic loss due to sickness . . . a very serious matter for many families with and without incomes, and therefore, an unfair burden upon the medical profession.
Franklin D. Roosevelt (1882–1945) US Democratic President.
Address on the Problems of Economic and Social Security, 14 Nov 1934

HEALTHY EATING
See also **HEALTHY LIVING.**

1   Diet cures more than the lancet.
    Anonymous

2   A good Kitchen is a good Apothicaries shop.
    William Bullein (d. 1576)
    The Bulwark Against All Sickness

3   One should eat to live, not live to eat.
    Cicero (106 BC–43 BC) Roman orator and statesman.
    Rhetoricorum, LV

4   Gluttony is an emotional escape, a sign something is eating us.
    Peter de Vries (1906–) US writer.
    Comfort Me with Apples, Ch. 15

5   Doctors are always working to preserve our health and cooks to destroy it,
    but the latter are the more often successful.
    Denis Diderot (1713–84) French philosopher and writer.

6   First need in the reform of hospital management? That's easy! The death of
    all dietitians, and the resurrection of a French chef.
    Martin H. Fischer (1879–1962)
    Fischerisms (Howard Fabing and Ray Marr)

7   I eat to live, to serve, and also, if it so happens, to enjoy, but I do not eat
    for the sake of enjoyment.
    Mahatma Gandhi (Mohandas Karamchand Gandhi; 1869–1948) Indian national
    leader.
    Attrib.

8   He that eats till he is sick must fast till he is well.
    Hebrew proverb

9   Food is so fundamental, more so than sexuality, aggression, or learning, that
    it is astounding to realize the neglect of food and eating in depth psychology.
    James Hillman
    Womansize (Kim Chernin)

10 One swears by wholemeal bread, one by sour milk; vegetarianism is the only
    road to salvation of some, others insist not only on vegetables alone, but on
    eating those raw. At one time the only thing that matters is calories; at an-
    other time they are crazy about vitamins or about roughage.
    The scientific truth may be put quite briefly; eat moderately, having an ordi-
    nary mixed diet, and don't worry.
    Sir Robert Hutchison (1871–1960)
    Newcastle Medical Journal, Vol. 12, 1932

11 Fasting is a medicine.
    St. John Chrysostom (c. 345–407) Bishop of Constantinopole and Doctor of
    the Church.
    Homilies on the Statutes, III

12   Food is an important part of a balanced diet.
     Fran Lebowitz (1950–   ) US writer.
     Metropolitan Life, 'Food for Thought and Vice Versa'

13   I told my doctor I get very tired when I go on a diet, so he gave me pep
     pills. Know what happened? I ate faster.
     Joe E. Lewis

14   The Chinese do not draw any distinction between food and medicine.
     Lin Yutang (1895–   )
     The Importance of Living, Ch. 9, Sect. 7

15   One should eat to live, not live to eat.
     Molière (Jean-Baptiste Poquelin; 1622–73) French dramatist.
     L'Avare, III:5

16   Some breakfast food manufacturer hit upon the simple notion of emptying out
     the leavings of carthorse nosebags, adding a few other things like unconsumed
     portions of chicken layer's mash, and the sweepings of racing stables, packing
     the mixture in little bags and selling them in health food shops.
     Frank Muir (1920–   ) British writer and broadcaster.
     Upon My Word!

17   Diet away your stress, tension and anxiety; a new commonsense plan for the
     control of low blood sugar related disorders, including overeating and obesity,
     migraine headaches, alcoholism, mental disturbances, hypoglycaemia and
     hyperactivity.
     J. Daniel Palm
     Extract from book cover by J. Daniel Palm, 1976

18   A little with quiet is the only diet.
     Proverb

19   An apple a day keeps the doctor away.
     Proverb

20   There are millions of vegetarians in the world but only one Bernard Shaw.
     You do not obtain eminence quite so cheaply as by eating macaroni instead
     of mutton chops.
     George Bernard Shaw (1856–1950) Irish dramatist and critic.
     Replying to a suggestion, during the meat shortage of the 1914–18 war, that
     he should be cited as an example of the advantages of vegetarianism

21   A man of my spiritual intensity does not eat corpses.
     George Bernard Shaw
     Attrib.

22   The thought of two thousand people crunching celery at the same time horri-
     fied me.
     George Bernard Shaw
     The Greatest Laughs of All Time (G. Lieberman)

Explaining why he had turned down an invitation to a vegetarian gala dinner

23 Better lose a supper than have a hundred physicians.
    Spanish proverb

24 Kitchen Physic is the best Physic.
    Jonathan Swift (1667–1745) Anglo-Irish priest, poet, and satirist.
    Polite Conversation, Dialogue II

25 The proverb warns that, 'You should not bite the hand that feeds you.' But
    maybe you should, if it prevents you from feeding yourself.
    Thomas Szasz (1920–) US psychiatrist.
    The Second Sin, 'Control and Self-control'

26 Illness isn't the only thing that spoils the appetite.
    Ivan Turgenev (1818–83) Russian novelist and dramatist.
    A Month in the Country, IV

27 A food is not necessarily essential just because your child hates it.
    Katherine Whitehorn (1926–) British journalist.
    How to Survive Children

28 It was my Uncle George who discovered that alcohol was a food well in ad-
    vance of modern medical thought.
    P. G. Wodehouse (1881–1975) British-born US humorous writer.
    The Inimitable Jeeves, Ch. 16

HEALTHY LIVING
See also **EXERCISE, HEALTHY EATING, HYGIENE.**

1 Why, Madam, do you know there are upward of thirty yards of bowels
   squeezed underneath that girdle of your daughter's? Go home and cut it; let
   Nature have fair play, and you will have no need of my advice.
   John Abernethy (1764–1831) English surgeon.
   Memoirs of John Abernethy, Ch. 33 (George Macilwain)
   Advice to a lady who took her tightly laced daughter to him

2 Health and cheerfulness mutually beget each other.
   Joseph Addison (1672–1719) English essayist.
   The Spectator, no. 387

3 Irritations of the eyes, which are caused by smoke, over-heating, dust, or sim-
   ilar injury, are easy to heal; the patient being advised first of all to avoid the
   irritating causes; . . . For the disease ceases without the use of any kind of
   medicine, if only a proper way of living be adopted.
   Aetios (c. 535)
   Tetrabiblon, Sermo II

4   Who lives medically lives miserably.
    Anonymous
    Anatomy of Melancholy (Robert Burton)

5   Get up at five, have lunch at nine,
    Supper at five, retire at nine.
    And you will live to ninety-nine.
    Anonymous
    Works, Bk. IV, Ch. 64 (François Rabelais)

6   A faithful friend is the medicine of life.
    Bible: Ecclesiasticus
    6:16

7   I answer 20 000 letters a year and so many couples are having problems be-
    cause they are not getting the right proteins and vitamins.
    Barbara Cartland (1902–) British romantic novelist.
    The Observer, 'Sayings of the Week', 31 Aug 1986

8   To avoid sickness, eat less, to prolong life, worry less.
    Chu Hui Weng
    Bulletin of the New York Academy of Medicine, 4:985, 1928 (F.H. Garrison)

9   Exercise and temperance can preserve something of our early strength even in
    old age.
    Cicero (106 BC–43 BC) Roman orator and statesman.
    An Old Age, X

10 The strongest possible piece of advice I would give to any young woman is:
    Don't screw around, and don't smoke.
    Edwina Currie (1946–) British politician.
    The Observer, 'Sayings of the Week', 3 Apr 1988

11 Fresh air impoverishes the doctor.
    Danish proverb

12 Eat not to dullness; drink not to elevation.
    Benjamin Franklin (1706–90) US scientist and statesman.
    Autobiography, Ch. 5

13 The disease of an evil conscience is beyond the practice of all the physicians
    of all the countries in the world.
    William E. Gladstone (1809–98)
    Speech, Plumstead, 1878

14 Healthy people are those who live in healthy homes on a healthy diet; in an
    environment equally fit for birth, growth, work, healing, and dying . . .
    Healthy people need no bureaucratic interference to mate, give birth, share
    the human condition and die.
    Ivan Illich (1926–) Austrian sociologist.
    Medical Nemesis

15 The healthy die first.
Italian proverb

16 The deviation of man from the state in which he was originally placed by nature seems to have proved to him a prolific source of diseases.
Edward Jenner (1749–1823) English physician.
An Inquiry into the Causes and Effects of the Variolae Vaccinae, or Cow-Pox

17 Your prayer must be for a sound mind in a sound body.
Juvenal (Decimus Junius Juvenalis; c. 60 AD–130 AD) Roman satirist.
Satires, X

18 What have I gained by health? intolerable dullness. What by early hours and moderate meals?–a total blank.
Charles Lamb (1775–1834) British essayist.
Letter to William Wordsworth, 22 Jan 1830

19 Joy and Temperance and Repose
Slam the door on the doctor's nose.
Henry Wadsworth Longfellow (1807–82) US poet.
The Sinngedichte of Friedrich von Logau

20 Medicine is a collection of uncertain prescriptions, the results of which, taken collectively, are more fatal than useful to mankind. Water, air, and cleanliness are the chief articles in my pharmacopoeia.
Napoleon I (Napoleon Bonaparte; 1769–1821) French emperor.

21 Patients should have rest, food, fresh air, and exercise – the quadrangle of health.
Sir William Osler (1849–1919) Canadian physician.
Sir William Osler: Aphorisms, Ch. 3 (William B. Bean)

22 The best of healers is good cheer.
Pindar (518 BC–438 BC) Greek poet.
Nemean Ode, IV

23 A man ought to handle his body like the sail of a ship, and neither lower and reduce it much when no cloud is in sight, nor be slack and careless in managing it when he comes to suspect something is wrong.
Plutarch (c. 46–c. 120) Greek biographer and essayist.
Moralia, 'Advice about Keeping Well'

24 An apple a day keeps the doctor away.
Proverb

25 Eat and drink measurely, and defy the mediciners.
Proverb

26 Use your health even to the point of wearing it out. That is what it is for. Spend all you have before you die, and do not outlive yourself.
George Bernard Shaw (1856–1950) Irish dramatist and critic.
The Doctor's Dilemma, 'Preface on Doctors'

27 When you are so poor that you cannot afford to refuse eighteenpence from a man who is too poor to pay you any more, it is useless to tell him that what he or his sick child needs is not medicine, but more leisure, better clothes, better food, and a better drained and ventilated house.
George Bernard Shaw
The Doctor's Dilemma, 'Preface on Doctors'

28 Living well and beautifully and justly are all one thing.
Socrates (469 BC–399 BC) Greek philosopher.
Crito (Plato)

29 I live in a constant endeavour to fence against the infirmities of ill health, and other evils of life, by mirth.
Laurence Sterne (1713–68) Irish-born English writer and churchman.
Tristram Shandy, Dedication

30 The twentieth century will be remembered chiefly, not as an age of political conflicts and technical inventions, but as an age in which human society dared to think of the health of the whole human race as a practical objective.
Arnold Toynbee (1889–1975) British historian.

31 Regimen is superior to medicine.
Voltaire (François-Marie Arouet; 1694–1778) French writer and philosopher.
A Philosophical Dictionary, 'Physicians'

32 I think it must be so, for I have been drinking it for sixty-five years and I am not dead yet.
Voltaire
Attrib.
On learning that coffee was considered a slow poison

HEART

1 When I first gave my mind to vivisection, as a means of discovering the motions and uses of the heart, and sought to discover these from actual inspection, and not from the writings of others, I found the task so truly arduous, so full of difficulties, that I was almost tempted to think with Fracastorius, that the motion of the heart was only to be comprehended by God.
William Harvey (1578–1657) English physician and anatomist.
On the Motion of the Heart and Blood in Animals, Ch. 1

HERBALISM

1   Why should a man die who has sage in his garden?
    Anonymous
    Regimen Sanitatis, Salernitanum

2   The Lord hath created medicines out of the earth; and he that is wise will
    not abhor them.
    Bible: Ecclesiasticus
    38:4

3   The spectacular advances made in therapeutics by industry during recent years
    tend to make us forget the medicinal value of plants. Their usefulness is far
    from negligible; their active principles are manifold and well-balanced.
    Dr. Paul Fruictier
    Grandmother's Secrets (Jean Palaiseul)

4   Anything green that grew out of the mould
    Was an excellent herb to our fathers of old.
    Rudyard Kipling (1865–1936) Indian-born British writer.
    Grandmother's Secrets (Jean Palaiseul)

5   Learn from the beasts the physic of the field.
    Alexander Pope (1688–1744) English poet.
    Essay on Man

6   O mickle is the powerful grace that lies in herbs plants, stones and their true
    qualities.
    William Shakespeare (1564–1616) English dramatist and poet.
    Romeo and Juliet, II

7   He preferred to know the power of herbs and their value for curing purposes,
    and, heedless of glory, to exercise that quiet art.
    Virgil (Publius Vergilius Maro; 70 BC–19 BC) Roman poet.
    Aeneid

HEREDITY

1   The law of heredity is that all undesirable traits come from the other parent.
    Anonymous

2   A person may be indebted for a nose or an eye, for a graceful carriage or a
    voluble discourse, to a great-aunt or uncle, whose existence he has scarcely
    heard of.
    William Hazlitt (1778–1830) British essayist.
    On Personal Character

3   Our humanity rests upon a series of learned behaviors, woven together into
    patterns that are infinitely fragile and never directly inherited.
    Margaret Mead (1901–78) US anthropologist.
    Male and Female, Ch. 9

4   Talent is hereditary; it may be the common possession of a whole family
    (e.g., the Bach family); genius is not transmitted; it is never diffused, but is
    strictly individual.
    Otto Weininger (1880–1903)
    Sex and Character, Pt. II, Ch. 4

HISTORY OF MEDICINE

1   If the science of medicine is not to be lowered to the rank of a mere
    mechanical profession it must pre-occupy itself with its history. The pursuit of
    the development of the human mind, this is the role of the historian.
    Emile Littré (1801–81)

2   The history of medicine does not depart from the history of the people.
    James G. Mumford (1863–1914)

3   The first cry of pain through the primitive jungle was the first call for a phy-
    sician . . . Medicine is a natural art, conceived in sympathy and born of ne-
    cessity; from instinctive procedures developed the specialized science that is
    practised today.
    Victor Robinson (1886–1947)
    The Story of Medicine

4   After twenty years one is no longer quoted in the medical literature. Every
    twenty years one sees a republication of the same ideas.
    Béla Schick (1877–1967) Austrian pediatrician.
    Aphorisms and Facetiae of Béla Schick, 'Early Years' (I.J. Wolf)

5   The very popular hunting for 'Fathers' of every branch of medicine and every
    treatment is, therefore, rather foolish; it is unfair not only to the mothers and
    ancestors but also to the obstetricians and midwives.
    Henry E. Sigerist (1891–1957)
    A History of Medicine, Vol. I, Introduction

6   The history of medicine is a story of amazing foolishness and amazing
    intelligence.
    Jerome Tarshis

HOLISTIC MEDICINE

1   A careful physician . . . , before he attempts to administer a remedy to his pa-

tient, must investigate not only the malady of the man he wishes to cure, but also his habits when in health, and his physical constitution.
Cicero (106 BC–43 BC) Roman orator and statesman.
On the Orator, II

2   A physician is obligated to consider more than a diseased organ, more even than the whole man – he must view the man in his world.
Harvey Cushing (1869–1939) US surgeon.
Man Adapting, Ch. 12 (René J. Dubos)

3   Natural forces are the healers of disease.
Hippocrates (c. 460 BC–c. 377 BC) Greek physician.
Epidemics, VI

4   When the minds of the people are closed and wisdom is locked out they remain tied to disease. Yet their feelings and desires should be investigated and made known, their wishes and ideas should be followed; and then it becomes apparent that those who have attained spirit and energy are flourishing and prosperous, while those perish who lose their spirit and energy.
Huang Ti (The Yellow Emperor; 2697 BC–2597 BC)
Nei Ching Su Wên, Bk. 4, Sect. 13

5   Knowledge indeed is a desirable, a lovely possession, but I do not scruple to say that health is more so. It is of little consequence to store the mind with science if the body be permitted to become debilitated. If the body be feeble, the mind will not be strong.
Thomas Jefferson (1743–1826) US statesman.
Letter to Thomas M. Randolph, Jr., 27 Aug 1786

6   Are you sick, or are you sullen?
Samuel Johnson (1709–84) English lexicographer and writer.
Letter to James Boswell, 5 Nov 1784

7   Heavy thoughts bring on physical maladies; when the soul is oppressed so is the body.
Martin Luther (1483–1546) German Protestant reformer.
Table-Talk, 'Of Temptation and Tribulation'

8   Body and soul cannot be separated for purposes of treatment, for they are one and indivisible. Sick minds must be healed as well as sick bodies.
C. Jeff Miller (1874–1936)
Surgery, Gynecology & Obstetrics, 52:488, 1931

9   The cure of many diseases is unknown to the physicians of Hellas, because they are ignorant of the whole, which ought to be studied also; for the part can never be well unless the whole is well. . . . This is the great error of our day in the treatment of the human body, that the physicians separate the soul from the body.
Plato (c. 427 BC–347 BC) Greek philosopher.
Charmides

10 Well in body
    But sick in mind.
    Plautus (c. 254 BC–c. 184 BC) Roman dramatist.
    Epidicus, I:2

11 The body must be repaired and supported, if we would preserve the mind in
    all its vigour.
    Pliny the Younger (Gaius Plinius Caecilius Secundus; c. 62 AD–c. 113 AD)
    Epistles, I, 9

12 The human body is like a bakery with a thousand windows. We are looking
    into only one window of the bakery when we are investigating one particular
    aspect of a disease.
    Béla Schick (1877–1967) Austrian pediatrician.
    Aphorisms and Facetiae of Béla Schick, 'Early Years' (I. J. Wolf)

13 Disease has social as well as physical, chemical, and biological causes.
    Henry E. Siegrist (1891–1957)

HOMEOPATHY

1 HOMEOPATHY, n. A school of medicine midway between Allopathy and
   Christian Science. To the last both the others are distinctly inferior, for
   Christian Science will cure imaginary diseases, and they can not.
   Ambrose Bierce (1842–c. 1914) US writer and journalist.
   The Devil's Dictionary

2 Homeopathy is insignificant as an act of healing, but of great value as criti-
   cism on the hygeia or medical practice of the time.
   Ralph Waldo Emerson (1803–82) US poet and essayist.
   Essays (Second Series), 'Nominalist and Realist'

3 Like cures like.
   Samuel Hahnemann (1755–1843) German physician, founder of homeopathy.
   Motto for homeopathy
   Also attributed to Hippocrates.

4 By opposites opposites are cured.
   Hippocrates (c. 460 BC–c. 377 BC) Greek physician.
   Deflatibus, Vol. I

5 Homeopathy . . . a mingled mass of perverse ingenuity, of tinsel erudition,
   of imbecile credulity, and of artful misrepresentation, too often mingled in
   practice . . . with heartless and shameless imposition.
   Oliver Wendell Holmes (1809–94) US writer and physician.
   Medical Essays, 'Homeopathy and Its Kindred Delusions'

6 So long as the body is affected through the mind, no audacious device, even

of the most manifestly dishonest character, can fail of producing occasional good to those who yield it an implicit or even a partial faith.
Oliver Wendell Holmes
Medical Essays, 'Homoeopathy and its Kindred Delusions'

HOMOSEXUALITY

1   But the men of Sodom were wicked and sinners before the Lord exceedingly.
Bible: Genesis
13:13

2   I am the Love that dare not speak its name.
Lord Alfred Douglas (1870–1945) British writer and poet.
Two Loves

3   This sort of thing may be tolerated by the French, but we are British – thank God.
Lord Montgomery (1887–1976) British field marshal.
Daily Mail, 27 May 1965
Comment on a bill to relax the laws against homosexuals

4   If Michelangelo had been straight, the Sistine Chapel would have been wallpapered.
Robin Tyler US comedienne.
Speech to gay-rights rally, Washington, 9 Jan 1988

HOPE

1   He that lives upon hope will die fasting.
Benjamin Franklin (1706–90) US scientist and statesman.
The Way to Wealth

2   Confidence and hope do be more good than physic.
Galen (fl. 2nd century) Greek physician.

3   Death is the greatest evil, because it cuts off hope.
William Hazlitt (1778–1830) British essayist and journalist.
Characteristics, 35

4   Hope is the physician of each misery.
Irish proverb

5   Hope is necessary in every condition. The miseries of poverty, sickness, of captivity, would, without this comfort, be insupportable.
Samuel Johnson (1709–84) English lexicographer and writer.
The Rambler, 67

6   The first qualification for a physician is hopefulness.
James Little (1836–85)

7   Always give the patient hope, even when death seems at hand.
    Ambroise Paré (c. 1517–90)

8   While there's life there's hope.
    Proverb

9   The miserable have no other medicine.
    But only hope.
    William Shakespeare (1564–1616) English dramatist and poet.
    Measure for Measure, III:1

10 The doctor says there is no hope, and as he does the killing he ought to
    know.
    Gaspar Zavala y Zamora (d. 1813)
    El Triunfo del Amor y de la Amistad, II:8

HOSPITALS
See also **NURSING.**

1   So it was all modern and scientific and well-arranged. You could die very
    nearly as privately in a modern hospital as you could in the Grand Central
    Station, and with much better care.
    Stephen Vincent Benét (1898–1943) US writer.
    Tales of Our Time, 'No Visitors'

2   Our hospital organization has grown up with no plan, with no system; it is
    unevenly distributed over the country . . . I would rather be kept alive in the
    efficient if cold altruism of a large hospital than expire in a gush of warm
    sympathy in a small one.
    Aneurin Bevan (1897–1960) British Labour politician.
    Speech, House of Commons, 30 Apr 1946
    Introducing the National Health Service Bill

3   It has been considered from the point of view of the hygienist, the physician,
    the architect, the tax-payer, the superintendents, and the nurse, but of the
    several hundred books, pamphlets, and articles on the subject with which I
    am acquainted, I do not remember to have seen one from the point of view
    of the patient.
    John Shaw Billings (1838–1913)
    Public Health Reports, 2:384, 1874–75

4   I believe it is most certainly possible to design features in such buildings that
    are positively healing; for instance I believe that courtyards, colonnades, and
    running water are healing features. It can't be easy to be healed in a soulless
    concrete box, with characterless windows, in hospitable corridors, and purely
    functional wards. The spirit needs healing as well as the body.
    Charles, Prince of Wales (1948–) Eldest son of Elizabeth II.
    Television documentary, 1988

5   One of the most difficult things to contend with in a hospital is the assump-
    tion on the part of the staff that because you have lost your gall bladder you
    have also lost your mind.
    Jean Kerr (1923–) US dramatist, screenwriter, and humorist.
    Please Don't Eat the Daisies, 'Operation Operation'

6   The ultimate indignity is to be given a bedpan by a stranger who calls you by
    your first name.
    Maggie Kuhn (1905–) US writer and social activist.
    The Observer, 20 Aug 1978

7   If you are hidebound with prejudice, if your temper is sentimental, you can
    go through the wards of a hospital and be as ignorant of man at the end as
    you were at the beginning.
    W. Somerset Maugham (1874–1965) British novelist and doctor.
    The Summing Up

8   The sooner patients can be removed from the depressing influence of general
    hospital life the more rapid their convalescence.
    Charles H. Mayo (1865–1939) US physician.
    Journal-Lancet, 36:1, 1916

9   'She says, if you please, sir, she only wants to be let die in peace.'
    'What! and the whole class to be disappointed, impossible! Tell her she can't
    be allowed to die in peace; it is against the rules of the hospital!'
    John Fisher Murray (1811–65)
    The World of London

10 It may seem a strange principle to enunciate as the very first requirement in a
    Hospital that it should do the sick no harm.
    Florence Nightingale (1820–1910) British nurse.
    Notes on Hospitals, Preface

11 That should assure us of at least 45 minutes of undisturbed privacy.
    Dorothy Parker (1893–1967) US writer and wit.
    The Algonquin Wits (R. Drennan)
    In hospital, pressing the bell for the nurse

12 Here, at whatever hour you come, you will find light and help and human
    kindness.
    Albert Schweitzer (1875–1965) French Protestant theologian, philosopher, and
    physician.
    Inscribed on the lamp outside his jungle hospital at Lambaréné

HUMAN CONDITION

1   Man that is born of a woman is of few days, and full of trouble.
    Bible: Job
    14:1

2 The human race, to which so many of my readers belong.
   G. K. Chesterton (1874–1936) British writer.
   The Napoleon of Notting Hill, Vol. I, Ch. 1

3 Fade far away, dissolve, and quite forget
   What thou among the leaves hast never known,
   The weariness, the fever, and the fret,
   Here, where men sit and hear each other groan.
   John Keats (1795–1821) British poet.
   Ode to a Nightingale

4 Brief and powerless is Man's life; on him and all his race the slow, sure doom
   falls pitiless and dark.
   Bertrand Russell (1872–1970) British philosopher.
   Mysticism and Logic, 'A Free Man's Worship'

HUMAN NATURE

1 A person seldom falls sick, but the bystanders are animated with a faint hope
   that he will die.
   Ralph Waldo Emerson (1803–82) US poet and essayist.
   Conduct of Life, 'Considerations by the Way'

HYGIENE
   See also **HEALTHY LIVING.**

1 Half of the secret of resistance to disease is cleanliness; the other half is
   dirtiness.
   Anonymous

2 Bath twice a day to be really clean, once a day to be passably clean, once a
   week to avoid being a public menace.
   Anthony Burgess (John Burgess Wilson; 1917–) British novelist.
   Mr. Enderby, Pt. I, Ch. 2

3 Man does not live by soap alone, and hygiene, or even health, is not much
   good unless you can take a healthy view of it – or, better still, feel a healthy
   indifference to it.
   G. K. Chesterton (1874–1936) British writer.
   All I Survey, 'On St. George Revivified'

4 Bathe early every day and sickness will avoid you.
   Indian (Hindustani) proverb

5 Hygiene is the corruption of medicine by morality. It is impossible to find a

hygienist who does not debase his theory of the healthful with a theory of the virtuous.
H. L. Mencken (1880–1956) US journalist and editor.
Prejudices, 'Types of Men'

6   What separates two people most profoundly is a different sense and degree of cleanliness.
Friedrich Nietzsche (1844–1900) German philosopher.
Beyond Good and Evil, 271

7   The first possibility of rural cleanliness lies in *water supply*.
Florence Nightingale (1820–1910) British nurse.
Letter to Medical Officer of Health, Nov 1891

8   Wash your hands often, your feet seldom, and your head never.
Proverb

9   Cleanliness is next to Godliness.
Proverb

HYPOCHONDRIA

1   A story circulated about a man who had decided gradually to give up every-thing that scientists have linked to cancer.
The first week, he cut out smoked fish and charcoal steaks.
The second week, he cut out smoking.
The third week, he cut out having relations with women.
The fourth week, he cut out drinking.
The fifth week, he cut out paper dolls.
Anonymous
The Boston Herald, 4 Sept 1965

2   I only take money from sick people.
Pierre Bretonneau (1778–1862)
Bulletin of the New York Academy of Medicine, 5:154, 1929
Comment to a hypochondriac

3   Hypochondriacs squander large sums of time in search of nostrums by which they vainly hope they may get more time to squander.
Charles C. Colton (1780–1832) British churchman and writer.
Lacon, 2

4   Nothing is more fatal to *Health*, than an *over Care* of it.
Benjamin Franklin (1706–90) US statesman and scientist.
Poor Richard's Almanack, 1760

5 If man thinks about his physical or moral state he usually discovers that he is
   ill.
   Johann Wolfgang von Goethe (1749–1832) German poet, dramatist and
   scientist.
   Sprüche in Prosa, Pt. I, Bk. II

6 This state I call the hypochondriac affection in men, and the hysteric in
   women . . . is a sort of walking dream, which, though a person be otherwise
   in sound health, makes him feel symptoms of every disease; and, though in-
   nocent, yet fills his mind with the blackest horrors of guilt.
   William Heberden (1710–1801)
   Commentaries on the History and Cure of Diseases, Ch. 49

7 Hungry Joe collected lists of fatal diseases and arranged them in alphabetical
   order so that he could put his finger without delay on any one he wanted to
   worry about.
   Joseph Heller (1923–   ) US novelist.
   Catch-22, Ch. 17

8 I never read a patent medicine advertisement without being impelled to the
   conclusion that I am suffering from the particular disease therein dealt with
   in its most virulent form.
   Jerome K. Jerome (1859–1927) British humorous writer.
   Three Men in a Boat, Ch. 1

9 Dear Doctor (said he one day to a common acquaintance, who lamented the
   tender state of his *inside*), do not be like the spider, man; and spin conversation thus incessantly out of thy own bowels.
   Samuel Johnson (1709–84) English lexicographer and writer.
   Johnsonian Miscellanies, Vol. I, 'Recollections of Dr. Johnson by Miss Reyn-
   olds' (G. B. Hill)

10 How sickness enlarges the dimensions of a man's self to himself.
   Charles Lamb (1775–1834) British essayist.
   Last Essays of Elia, 'The Convalescent'

11 Attention to health is the greatest hindrance to life.
   Plato (428 BC–347 BC) Greek philosopher.

12 He that is uneasy at every little pain is never without some ache.
   Proverb

13 Hypochondria torments us not only with causeless irritation with the things
   of the present; not only with groundless anxiety on the score of future misfor-
   tunes entirely of our own manufacture; but also with unmerited self-reproach
   for our own past actions.
   Arthur Schopenhauer (1788–1860) German philosopher.
   Parerga und Paralipomena, Vol. II, Ch. 26

14 Illness is the night-side of life, a more onerous citizenship. Everyone who is

born holds dual citizenship, in the kingdom of the well and in the kingdom
of the sick. Although we all prefer to use only the good passport, sooner or
later each of us is obliged, at least for a spell, to identify ourselves as citizens
of that other place.
Susan Sontag (1933–) US novelist and essayist.
Illness as Metaphor

15 People who are always taking care of their health are like misers, who are
hoarding a treasure which they have never spirit enough to enjoy.
Laurence Sterne (1713–68) Irish-born English writer and churchman.

16 He destroys his health by labouring to preserve it.
Virgil (Publius Vergilius Maro; 70 BC–19 BC) Roman poet.
Aeneid, Bk. XII

17 The imaginary complaints of indestructible old ladies.
E. B. White (1899–) US journalist and humorous writer.
Harper's Magazine, Nov 1941

18 An imaginary ailment is worse than a disease.
Yiddish proverb

I

ILLNESS
See also **DISEASE.**

1   I inhabit a weak, frail, decayed tenement; battered by the winds and broken
    in on by the storms, and, from all I can learn, the landlord does not intend
    to repair.
    John Quincy Adams (1767–1848) US statesman.
    Attrib.
    Said during his last illness

2   Be not slow to visit the sick: for that shall make thee to be beloved.
    Bible: Ecclesiasticus
    7:35

3   They that be whole need not a physician, but they that are sick.
    Bible: Matthew
    9:12

4   I reckon being ill as one of the greatest pleasures of life, provided one is not
    too ill and is not obliged to work till one is better.
    Samuel Butler (1835–1902) British writer.
    The Way of All Flesh, Ch. 80

5   As *sickness* is the greatest misery so the greatest misery of sickness is *solitude*.
    Solitude is a torment which is not threatened in *hell* itselfe.
    John Donne (1573–1631) English poet.
    Awakenings (Oliver W. Sacks)

6   To be too conscious is an illness – a real thorough-going illness.
    Fyodor Mikhailovich Dostoevsky (1821–81) Russian writer.
    Notes from Underground, 1

7   It is dainty to be sick if you have leisure and convenience for it.
    Ralph Waldo Emerson (1803–82) US poet and essayist.
    Journals, Vol. V

8   The multitude of the sick shall not make us deny the existence of health.
    Ralph Waldo Emerson
    The Conduct of Life, 'Worship'

9   A weary thing is sickness and its pains!
    Euripides (484 BC–406 BC) Greek dramatist.
    Hippolytus, 176

10   Much of the world's work is done by men who do not feel quite well. Marx
     is a case in point.
     J. K. Galbraith (1908–) US economist.
     The Age of Uncertainty

11   Illness makes a man a scoundrel.
     Samuel Johnson (1709–84) English lexicographer and writer.
     Letter to Fanny Burney, Jan 1788

12   To be sick is to enjoy monarchal prerogatives.
     Charles Lamb (1775–1834) English essayist and critic.
     Last Essays of Elia, 'The Convalescent'

13   How sickness enlarges the dimensions of a man's self to himself.
     Charles Lamb
     Last Essays of Elia, 'The Convalescent'

14   I am only half there when I am ill, and so there is only half a man to suffer.
     To suffer in one's whole self is so great a violation, that it is not to be
     endured.
     D. H. Lawrence (1885–1930) British writer.
     Letter to Catherine Carswell, 16 Apr 1916

15   The most important thing in illness is never to lose heart.
     Nikolai Lenin (Vladimir Ilyich Ulyanov; 1870–1924) Russian Communist leader.
     The Secret of Soviet Strength, Bk. II, Ch. 3, Sect. 2 (Hewlett Johnson)

16   Medicine makes sick patients, for doctors imagine diseases, as mathematics
     makes hypochondriacs and theology sinners.
     Martin Luther (1483–1546) German Protestant reformer.

17   One who is ill has not only the right but also the duty to seek medical aid.
     Maimonides (Moses ben Maimon; 1135–1204) Spanish-born Jewish philosopher
     and physician.

18   Illness is in part what the world has done to a victim, but in a larger part it
     is what the victim has done with his world, and with himself.
     Karl Menninger (1893–) US psychiatrist.
     Illness as Metaphor, Ch. 6 (Susan Sontag)

19   The sick are the greatest danger for the healthy; it is not from the strongest
     that harm comes to the strong, but from the weakest.
     Friedrich Nietzsche (1844–1900) German philosopher.
     Genealogy of Morals, Essay 3

20   Here am I dying of a hundred good symptoms.
     Alexander Pope (1688–1744) English poet.
     Said to George Lyttleton, 15 May 1744

21   He dies every day who lives a lingering life.
     Pierrard Poullet (fl. 1590)
     La Charité

22   Illness is the doctor to whom we pay most heed; to kindness, to knowledge,
     we make promise only, pain we obey.
     Marcel Proust (1871–1922) French writer.

23   Sickness is felt, but health not at all.
     Proverb

24   Sickness tells us what we are.
     Proverb

25   We are usually the best men when in the worst health.
     Proverb

26   Every man who feels well is a sick man neglecting himself.
     Jules Romains (1885–1972) French writer.
     Knock, ou le triomphe de la médecine

27   Illness is the night-side of life, a more onerous citizenship. Everyone who is
     born holds dual citizenship, in the kingdom of the well and in the kingdom
     of the sick. Although we all prefer to use only the good passport, sooner or
     later each of us is obliged, at least for a spell, to identify ourselves as citizens
     of the other place.
     Susan Sontag (1933–   ) US novelist and essayist.
     Illness as Metaphor

28   We are so fond of one another because our ailments are the same.
     Jonathan Swift (1667–1745) Anglo-Irish priest, poet, and satirist.
     Letter to Stella, 1 Feb 1711

29   Nor do I in any way approve of the modern sympathy with invalids. I con-
     sider it morbid. Illness of any kind is hardly a thing to be encouraged in
     others.
     Oscar Wilde (1856–1900) Irish-born British poet and dramatist.
     The Importance of Being Earnest, I

30   Considering how common illness is, how tremendous the spiritual change that
     it brings, how astonishing, when the lights of health go down, the undiscov-
     ered countries that are then disclosed, what wastes and deserts of the soul a
     slight attack of influenza brings to view, what precipices and lawns sprinkled
     with bright flowers a little rise of temperature reveals, what ancient and ob-
     durate oaks are uprooted in us by the act of sickness, how we go down into
     the pit of death and feel the waters of annihilation close above our heads and
     wake thinking to find ourselves in the presence of the angels and the harpers
     when we have a tooth out and come to the surface in the dentist's arm-chair
     and confuse his 'Rinse the mouth – rinse the mouth' with the greeting of the
     Deity stooping from the floor of Heaven to welcome us – when we think of

this, as we are so frequently forced to think of it, it becomes strange indeed that illness has not taken its place with love and battle and jealousy among the prime themes of literature.
Virginia Woolf (1882–1941) British writer.
The Moment and Other Essays, 'On Being Ill'

INCURABLE DISEASE

1   A good Doctor can foresee the fatal outcome of an incurable illness, when he cannot help, the experienced Doctor will take care not to aggravate the sick person's malady by tiring but injurious efforts; and in an impossible case he will not frustrate himself further with ineffective solicitude.
Hermann Boerhaave (1668–1738)
Atrocis, nec Descripti Prius, Morbi Historia

2   Not even remedies can master incurable diseases.
Seneca (c. 4 BC–65 AD) Roman writer and statesman.
Epistulae ad Lucilium

3   Even if the doctor does not give you a year, even if he hesitates about a month, make one brave push and see what can be accomplished in a week.
Robert Louis Stevenson (1850–94) Scottish writer.
Virginibus Puerisque, Ch. 5

INDIGESTION
See also **DIGESTION**.

1   Miss Davies has two expressions–joy and indigestion.
Anonymous
Referring to Marion Davies, US actress
Who Killed Society? (Cleveland Amory)

2   'Tis not *her* coldness, father,
That chills my labouring breast;
It's that confounded cucumber
I've eat and can't digest.
R. H. Barham ('Thomas Ingoldsby') (1788–1845) British humorous writer.
The Ingoldsby Legends, 'The Confession'

3   GLUTTON, n. A person who escapes the evils of moderation by committing dyspepsia.
Ambrose Bierce (1842–c. 1914) US writer and journalist.
The Devil's Dictionary

4   INDIGESTION, n. A disease which the patient and his friends frequently mistake for deep religious conviction and concern for the salvation of man-

kind. As the simple Red Man of the western wild put it, with, it must be confessed, a certain force: 'Plenty well, no pray; big bellyache, heap God.'
Ambrose Bierce
The Devil's Dictionary

5   I lead a most dyspeptic, solitary, self-shrouded *life*: consuming, if possible in silence, my considerable daily allotment of *pain*.
Thomas Carlyle (1795–1881) Scottish historian and essayist.
Letter to Ralph Waldo Emerson, 8 Feb 1839

6   To eat is human, to digest divine.
Charles T. Copeland (1860–1952)

7   Don't tell your friends about your indigestion:
'How are you!' is a greeting, not a question.
Arthur Guiterman
A Poet's Proverbs, 'Of Tact'

8   An indigestion is an excellent common-place for two people that never met before.
William Hazlitt (1788–1830) English essayist and journalist.
Literary Remains, 'The Fight'

9   Indigestion is charged by God with enforcing morality on the stomach.
Victor Hugo (1802–85) French poet, novelist, and dramatist.
Les Misérables, 'Fantine', Bk. III, Ch. 7

10 Many people think they have religion when they are troubled with dyspepsia.
Robert G. Ingersoll (1833–99) US lawyer and agnostic.
Liberty of Man, Woman and Child, Section 3

11 Confirmed dyspepsia is the apparatus of illusions.
George Meredith (1828–1909) British novelist.
The Ordeal of Richard Feverel

12 Drinking and sweating, – it's the life of a dyspeptic!
Seneca (c. 4 BC–65 AD) Roman writer and statesman.
Epistulae ad Lucilium, XV

13 He sows hurry and reaps indigestion.
Robert Louis Stevenson (1850–94) Scottish writer.
An Apology for Idlers

INSANITY
See **MENTAL ILLNESS.**

INSOMNIA
See also **SLEEP.**

1   It appears that every man's insomnia is as different from his neighbor's as are their daytime hopes and aspirations.
F. Scott Fitzgerald (1896–1940) US writer.
The Crack-up, 'Sleeping and Waking'

2   Insomnia never comes to a man who has to get up exactly at six o'clock. Insomnia troubles only those who can sleep any time.
Elbert G. Hubbard (1856–1915)
The Philistine, 'In Re Muldoon'

INVALIDS

1   Every invalid is a physician.
Irish proverb

2   The sick man is a parasite of society. In certain cases it is indecent to go on living. To continue to vegetate in a state of cowardly dependence upon doctors and special treatments, once the meaning of life, the right to life has been lost, ought to be regarded with the greatest contempt by society.
Friedrich Nietzsche (1844–1900) German philosopher.
The Twilight of the Idols, 'Skirmishes in a War with the Age'

J

JARGON

1   Nor bring to see me cease to live,
    Some doctor full of phrase and fame,
    To shake his sapient head, and give
    The ill he cannot cure a name.
    Matthew Arnold (1822–88) British poet and critic.
    'A Wish'

2   The modern haematologist, instead of describing in English what he can see,
    prefers to describe in Greek what he can't.
    Richard Asher (1912–   )
    Lancet, 2:359, 1959

3   Well I ask you? When you take your family on holiday, do you say 'I am tak-
    ing my gregarious egalitarian sibling group with me'?
    Richard Asher
    Lancet, 2:359, 1959

4   Medical men all over the world . . . merely entered into a tacit agreement to
    call all sorts of maladies people are liable to, in cold weather, by one name;
    so that one sort of treatment may serve for all, and their practice be thereby
    greatly simplified.
    Jane Welsh Carlyle (1801–66) The wife of Thomas Carlyle.
    Letter to John Welsh, 4 Mar 1837

5   Ad-i-ad-o-cho-kin-e-sis
    Is a term that will bolster my thesis
    That 'tis idle to seek
    Such precision in Greek
    When confusion it only increases.
    Horace B. and Ava C. English (1892–1961; fl. 20th century)
    A Comprehensive Dictionary of Psychological and Psychoanalytical Terms

6   When there is no explanation, they give it a name, which immediately ex-
    plains everything.
    Martin H. Fischer (1879–1962)
    Fischerisms (Howard Fabing and Ray Marr)

7   Whenever ideas fail, men invent words.
    Martin H. Fischer
    Fischerisms (Howard Fabing and Ray Marr)

8   You must learn to talk clearly. The jargon of scientific terminology which
    rolls off your tongues is mental garbage.
    Martin H. Fischer
    Fischerisms (Howard Fabing and Ray Marr)

9   The patient's ears remorseless he assails;
.   Murder with jargon where his medicine fails.
    Sir Samuel Garth (1661–1719) English physician and poet.
    The Dispensary

10 It is a distinct art to talk medicine in the language of the non-medical man.
    Edward H. Goodman (1879–   )

11 Some seventy years ago a promising young neurologist made a discovery that
    necessitated the addition of a new word to the English vocabulary. He in-
    sisted that this should be *knee-jerk*, and *knee-jerk* it has remained, in spite of
    the efforts of *patellar reflex* to dislodge it. He was my father; so perhaps I have
    inherited a prejudice in favour of home-made words.
    Sir Ernest Gowers (1880–1966)
    Plain Words, Ch. 5

12 The Spanish doctor who treated Yeats in Majorca reported to his Irish col-
    league. 'We have here an antique cardio-sclerotic of advanced years.' Gogarty
    tried to slur over the death sentence. 'Read it slowly and distinctly,' Yeats or-
    dered. He inclined his head. He followed the cadence with his finger. As the
    sound died away he exclaimed, 'Do you know, I would rather be called
    'Cardio-Sclerotic' than Lord of Lower Egypt.'
    T. R. Henn
    The Lonely Tower

13 I would never use a long word, even, where a short one would answer the
    purpose. I know there are professors in this country who 'ligate' arteries.
    Other surgeons only tie them, and it stops the bleeding just as well.
    Oliver Wendell Holmes (1809–94) US writer and physician.
    Medical Essays, 'Scholastic and Bedside Teaching'

14 Remember that even the learned ignorance of a nomenclature is something to
    have mastered, and may furnish pegs to hang facts upon which would other-
    wise have strewed the floor of memory in loose disorder.
    Oliver Wendell Holmes
    Medical Essays, 'The Young Practitioner'

15 There are things which will not be defined, and Fever is one of them. Be-
    sides, when a word had passed into everyday use, it is too late to lay a logical
    trap for its meaning, and think to apprehend it by a definition.
    Peter Mere Latham (1789–1875) US poet and essayist.
    General Remarks on the Practice of Medicine, Ch. 10, Pt. 1

16 The contraction of his obicular, the lateral obtusion of his sense centres, his
    night fears, his stomach trouble, the polyencephalitic condition of his youth,

and above all the heredity of his old father and young mother, combined to make him an hysterico-epileptic type, traceable in the paranoic psychoses evident in all he wrote.
Cesare Lombroso (1853–1909) Italian criminologist.
Referring to Emile Zola
Paris Was Yesterday (Janet Flanner)

17 There is no counting the names, that surgeons and anatomists give to the various parts of the human body . . . . I wonder whether mankind could not get along without all those names, which keep increasing every day, and hour, and moment. . . . But people seem to have a great love for names; for to know a great many names seems to look like knowing a good many things.
Herman Melville (1819–91) US novelist.
Redburn, Ch. 13

18 A man of true science . . . uses but few hard words, and those only when none other will answer his purpose; whereas the smatterer in science . . . thinks, that by mouthing hard words, he proves that he understands hard things.
Herman Melville
White Jacket, Ch. 63

19 They do certainly give very strange and new-fangled names to diseases.
Plato (c. 427 BC–347 BC) Greek philosopher.
Republic, III

20 The language of the men of medicine is a fearful concoction of sesquipedalian words, numbered by thousands.
Frederick Saunders (1807–1902)

21 People of wealth and rank never use ugly nakes for ugly things. Apoplexy is an affection of the head; paralysis is nervousness; gangrene is pain and inconvenience in the extremities.
Sydney Smith (1771–1845) British churchman, essayist and wit.
Letter to Mrs. Holland, Jan 1844

K

KINDNESS

1   Pleasant words are as an honeycomb, sweet to the soul, and health to the
    bones.
    Bible: Proverbs
    16:24

2   In the sick room, ten cents' worth of human understanding equals ten dollars'
    worth of medical science.
    Martin H. Fischer (1879–1962)
    Fischerisms (Howard Fabing and Ray Marr)

3   True kindness presupposes the faculty of imagining as one's own the suffering
    and joy of others.
    André Gide (1869–1951) French writer.

4   The natural dignity of our work, its unembarrassed kindness, its insight into
    life, its hold on science – for these privileges, and for all that they bring
    with them, up and up, high over the top of the tree, the very heavens open,
    preaching thankfulness.
    Stephen Paget (1855–1926)
    Confessio Medici, Epilogue

5   A word of kindness is better than a fat pie.
    Russian proverb

6   People pay the doctor for his trouble; for his kindness they still remain in his
    debt.
    Seneca (c. 4 BC–65 AD) Roman writer and statesman.

KNOWLEDGE

1   Teach thy tongue to say 'I do not know.'
    Maimonides (Moses ben Maimon; 1135–1204) Spanish-born Jewish philosopher
    and physician.

2   Sciences may be learned by rote, but Wisdom not.
    Laurence Sterne (1713–68) Irish-born English writer and churchman.
    Tristram Shandy

L

LAUGHTER

1 Laughter is the best medicine.
   Proverb

LIFE
   See also **HUMAN CONDITION, LIFE AND DEATH.**

1 A man of sixty has spent twenty years in bed and over three years eating.
   Arnold Bennett (1867–1931) British novelist.
   Bartlett's Unfamiliar Quotations (Leonard Louis Levinson)

2 Life is a partial, continuous, progressive, multiform and conditionally interactive self-realization of the potentialities of atomic electron states.
   John Desmond Bernal (1901–71)
   The Origin of Life

3 A faithful friend is the medicine of life.
   Bible: Ecclesiasticus
   6:16

4 Is life worth living? This is a question for an embryo, not for a man.
   Samuel Butler (1835–1902) British writer.

5 To live is like love, all reason is against it, and all healthy instinct for it.
   Samuel Butler
   Notebooks

6 Living is a sickness from which sleep provides relief every sixteen hours. It's a pallative. The remedy is death.
   Nicolas Chamfort (1741–94) French writer and wit.

7 Life is an incurable Disease.
   Abraham Cowley (1618–67) English poet.
   Pindarique Odes, 'To Dr. Scarborough', VI

8 Life was a funny thing that occurred on the way to the grave.
   Quentin Crisp (c. 1910–   ) British model, publicist, and writer.
   The Naked Civil Servant

9 Between
   Our birth and death we may touch understanding

As a moth brushes a window with its wing.
Christopher Fry (1907–) British dramatist.
The Boy with a Cart

10   Life is made up of sobs, sniffles and smiles, with sniffles predominating.
O. Henry (William Sydney Porter; 1862–1910) US writer.
The Gifts of the Magi

11   Life is a fatal complaint, and an eminently contagious one.
Oliver Wendell Holmes (1809–94) US writer and physician.
The Poet at the Breakfast Table, XII

12   Life is simply one damned thing after another.
Elbert Hubbard (1856–1915) US writer and editor.
Attrib.

13   The art of life is the avoiding of pain.
Thomas Jefferson (1743–1826) US statesman.
Bartlett's Unfamiliar Quotations (Leonard Louis Levinson)

14   Life is something to do when you can't get to sleep.
Fran Lebowitz (1950–) US writer.
The Observer, 21 Jan 1979

15   Life to me is like boarding-house wallpaper. It takes a long time to get used
to it, but when you finally do, you never notice that it's there. And then
you hear the decorators are arriving.
Derek Marlowe (1938–) British writer.
A Dandy in Aspic

16   It is not true that life is one damn thing after another—it's one damn thing
over and over.
Edna St. Vincent Millay (1892–1950) US poet.
Letters of Edna St. Vincent Millay

17   The aim of life is to live, and to live means to be aware, joyously, drunk-
enly, serenely, divinely aware.
Henry Miller (1891–1980) US novelist.
The Wisdom of the Heart, 'Creative Death'

18   Life is for each man a solitary cell whose walls are mirrors.
Eugene O'Neill (1888–1953) US dramatist.
Lazarus Laughed

19   Life is perhaps best regarded as a bad dream between two awakenings.
Eugene O'Neill
Marco Millions

20   Life is not a spectacle or a feast; it is a predicament.
George Santayana (1863–1952) Spanish-born US philosopher, poet, and critic.
Articles and Essays

21   There is no cure for birth and death save to enjoy the interval.
     George Santayana
     Soliloquies in England, 'War shrines'

22   It is only in the microscope that our life looks so big. It is an indivisible
     point, drawn out and magnified by the powerful lenses of Time and Space.
     Arthur Schopenhauer (1788–1860) German philosopher.
     Parerga and Paralipomena, 'The Vanity of Existence'

23   The purpose of human life is to serve and to show compassion and the will
     to help others.
     Albert Schweitzer (1875–1965) French Protestant theologian, philosopher, and
     physician.
     The Schweitzer Album

24   Life is a disease; and the only difference between one man and another is the
     stage of the disease at which he lives.
     George Bernard Shaw (1856–1950) Irish dramatist and critic.
     Back to Methuselah, II, 'Gospel of the Brothers Barnabas'

25   To preserve a man alive in the midst of so many chances and hostilities, is as
     great a miracle as to create him.
     Jeremy Taylor (1613–67) English Anglican theologian.
     Holy Dying

26   We begin to live when we have conceived life as a tragedy.
     W. B. Yeats (1865–1939) Irish poet.
     Autobiography

LIFE AND DEATH

1   The thing to remember is that each time of life has its appropriate rewards,
    whereas when you're dead it's hard to find the light switch. The chief prob-
    lem about death, incidentally, is the fear that there may be no afterlife – a
    depressing thought, particularly for those who have bothered to shave. Also,
    there is the fear that there is an afterlife but no one will know where it's be-
    ing held. On the plus side, death is one of the few things that can be done
    as easily lying down.
    Woody Allen (Allen Stewart Konigsberg; 1935–   ) US film actor and director.
    Without Feathers, 'The Early Essays'

2   Life, the permission to know death.
    Djuna Barnes (1892–   ) US writer.
    Nightwood

3   . . . Human life is mainly a process of filling in time until the arrival of

death, or Santa Claus, with very little choice, if any, of what kind of business one is going to transact during the long wait.
Eric Berne
Games People Play, Ch. 18

4   Life itself is but the shadow of death, and souls but the shadows of the living. All things fall under this name. The sun itself is but the dark *simulacrum*, and light but the shadow of God.
Sir Thomas Browne (1605–82) English physician and writer.
The Garden of Cyrus

5   Birth, and copulation, and death.
That's all the facts when you come to brass tacks.
T. S. Eliot (1888–1965) US-born British poet and dramatist.
Sweeney Agonistes, 'Fragment of an Agon'

6   The memory of birth and the expectation of death always lurk within the human being, making him separate from his fellows and consequently capable of intercourse with them.
E. M. Forster (1879–1970) British writer.
'What I Believe'

7   The most rational cure after all for the inordinate fear of death is to set a just value on life.
William Hazlitt (1778–1830) British essayist and journalist.
Table Talk, 'On the Fear of Death'

8   I believe that the struggle against death, the unconditional and self-willed determination to live, is the motive power behind the lives and activities of all outstanding men.
Hermann Hesse (1877–1962) German novelist and poet.
Steppenwolf, 'Treatise on the Steppenwolf'

9   Science says: 'We must live,' and seeks the means of prolonging, increasing, facilitating and amplifying life, of making it tolerable and acceptable; wisdom says: 'We must die,' and seeks how to make us die well.
Miguel de Unamuno y Jugo (1864–1936) Spanish writer and philosopher.
Essays and Soliloquies, 'Arbitrary Reflections'

10 There are only three events in a man's life; birth, life, and death; he is not conscious of being born, he dies in pain, and he forgets to live.
Jean de La Bruyère (1645–96) French writer and moralist.
Caractères

11 Many men would take the death-sentence without a whimper to escape the life-sentence which fate carries in her other hand.
T. E. Lawrence (1888–1935) British soldier and writer.
The Mint, I, Ch. 4

12   If you wish to live, you must first attend your own funeral.
     Katherine Mansfield (1888–1923) New-Zealand-born British writer.
     Katherine Mansfield (Antony Alpers)

13   Life is a great surprise. I do not see why death should not be an even greater
     one.
     Vladimir Nabokov (1899–1977) Russian-born US novelist.
     Pale Fire, 'Commentary'

14   Life levels all men: death reveals the eminent.
     George Bernard Shaw (1856–1950) Irish dramatist and critic.
     Maxims for Revolutionists

15   If we are aware of what indicates life, which everyone may be supposed to
     know, though perhaps no one can say that he truly and clearly understands
     what constitutes it, we at once arrive at the discrimination of death. It is the
     cessation of the phenomena with which we are so especially familiar–the
     phenomena of life.
     J. G. Smith
     Principles of Forensic Medicine

16   All say, 'How hard it is that we have to die' – a strange complaint to come
     from the mouths of people who have had to live.
     Mark Twain (Samuel L. Clemens; 1835–1910) US writer.
     Pudd'nhead Wilson

LIVER

1   LIVER, n. A large red organ thoughtfully provided by nature to be bilious
    with. . . . It was at one time considered the seat of life; hence its name –
    liver, the thing we live with.
    Ambrose Bierce (1842–c. 1914) US writer and journalist.
    The Devil's Dictionary

LONGEVITY

1   LONGEVITY, n. Uncommon extension of the fear of death.
    Ambrose Bierce (1842–c. 1914) US writer and journalist.
    The Devil's Dictionary

2   People always wonder how I have achieved such a ripe age, and I can only
    say I never felt the urge to partake of the grape, the grain, or the weed, but
    I do eat everything.
    Mrs. Mary Borah
    Bartlett's Unfamiliar Quotations (Leonard Louis Levinson)
    Said at the age of 100

3   There is no short-cut to longevity. To win it is the work of a lifetime, and the promotion of it is a branch of preventive medicine.
Sir James Crichton-Browne (1840–1938)
The Prevention of Senility

4   Have a chronic disease and take care of it.
Oliver Wendell Holmes (1809–94) US writer and physician.
His formula for longevity.

5   Life protracted is protracted woe.
Samuel Johnson (1709–84) English lexicographer and writer.
The Vanity of Human Wishes

6   Get your room full of good air, then shut up the windows and keep it. It will keep for years. Anyway, don't keep using your lungs all the time. Let them rest.
Stephen Leacock (1869–1944) English-born Canadian economist and humorist.
Literary Lapses, 'How to Live to be 200'

7   Do not try to live forever. You will not succeed.
George Bernard Shaw (1856–1950) Irish dramatist and critic.
The Doctor's Dilemma, 'Preface on Doctors'

8   I smoke almost constantly, sometimes in the middle of the night. And I drink anything I can get my hands on.
Joe Smart
Bartlett's Unfamiliar Quotations (Leonard Louis Levinson)
On his 100th birthday.

9   They live ill who expect to live always.
Publilius Syrus (1st century BC) Roman dramatist.
Moral Sayings, 457

10 Keep breathing.
Sophie Tucker (1884–1966) Russian-born US singer and vaudeville star.
Attrib.
Her reply, at the age of 80, when asked the secret of her longevity

M

MANKIND

1 Man, when perfected, is the best of animals, but, when separated from law
   and justice, he is the worst of all.
   Aristotle (384 BC–322 BC) Greek philosopher and scientist.
   Politics, 1

2 Is a man a salvage at heart, skinned o'er with fragile Manners? Or is
   salvagery but a faint taint in the natural man's gentility, which erupts now
   and again like pimples on an angel's arse?
   John Barth (1930–) US novelist and academic.
   The Sot-Weed Factor, 3

3 Drinking when we are not thirsty and making love all year round, madam;
   that is all there is to distinguish us from other animals.
   Beaumarchais (1732–99) French dramatist.
   Le Mariage de Figaro, II:21

4 And God said, Let us make man in our image, after our likeness: and let
   them have dominion over the fish of the sea, and over the fowl of the air,
   and over the cattle, and over all the earth, and over every creeping thing
   that creepeth upon the earth.
   So God created man in his own image, in the image of God created he him;
   male and female created he them.
   And God blessed them, and God said unto them, Be fruitful, and multiply,
   and replenish the earth, and subdue it: and have dominion over the fish of
   the sea, and over the fowl of the air, and over every living thing that
   moveth upon the earth.
   Bible: Genesis
   1:26–28

5 MAN, n. An animal so lost in rapturous contemplation of what he thinks he
   is as to overlook what he indubitably ought to be.
   Ambrose Bierce (1842–c. 1914) US writer and journalist.
   The Devil's Dictionary

6 What is man, when you come to think upon him, but a minutely set, ingenious machine for turning, with infinite artfulness, the red wine of Shiraz
   into urine?
   Karen Blixen (Isak Dinesen; 1885–1962) Danish writer.
   Seven Gothic Tales, 'The Dreamers'

7   The true science and the true study of man is man.
    Pierre Charron (1541–1603) French theologian and philosopher.
    Traité de la sagesse, Bk. I, Ch. 1

8   Man is an exception, whatever else he is. If he is not the image of God,
    then he is a disease of the dust.
    G. K. Chesterton (1874–1936) British writer.
    All Things Considered, 'Wine When It Is Red'

9   A wonderful fact to reflect upon, that every human creature is constituted to
    be that profound secret and mystery to every other.
    Charles Dickens (1812–70) British novelist.
    A Tale of Two Cities, 1

10 Man is physically as well as metaphysically a thing of shreds and patches,
    borrowed unequally from good and bad ancestors, and a misfit from the start.
    Ralph Waldo Emerson (1803–82) US poet and essayist.
    The Conduct of Life, 'Beauty'

11 Every man has a wild beast within him.
    Frederick the Great (1712–86) Prussian king.
    Letter to Voltaire, 1759

12 Man is Nature's sole mistake!
    W. S. Gilbert (1836–1922) British dramatist and comic writer.
    Princess Ida

13 Human beings are like timid punctuation marks sprinkled among the incom-
    prehensible sentences of life.
    Jean Giraudoux (1882–1944) French dramatist and writer.
    Siegfried, 2

14 Man is a mind betrayed, not served, by his organs.
    Edmond and Jules de Goncourt (1822–96; 1830–70) French writers.
    Journal, 30 July 1861

15 The human race will be the cancer of the planet.
    Sir Julian Huxley (1887–1975) British biologist.
    Attrib.

16 Man as we know him is a poor creature; but he is halfway between an ape
    and a god and he is travelling in the right direction.
    W. R. Inge (1860–1954) British churchman.
    Outspoken Essays: Second Series, 'Confessio Fidei'

17 I'll give you my opinion of the human race . . . Their heart's in the right
    place, but their head is a thoroughly inefficient organ.
    W. Somerset Maugham (1874–1965) British writer and doctor.
    The Summing Up

18   Man is a beautiful machine that works very badly. He is like a watch of
     which the most that can be said is that its cosmetic effect is good.
     H. L. Mencken (1880–1956) US journalist and editor.
     Minority Report, 20

19   Every man carries the entire form of human condition.
     Michel de Montaigne (1533–92) French essayist and moralist.
     Essays, 'Of repentance'

20   A human being, he wrote, is a whispering in the steam pipes on a cold
     night; dust sifted through a locked window; one or the other half of an un-
     solved equation; a pun made by God; an ingenious assembly of portable
     plumbing.
     Christopher Morley (1890–1957) US writer and journalist.
     Human Being, Ch. 11

21   There are one hundred and ninety-three living species of monkeys and apes.
     One hundred and ninety-two of them are covered with hair. The exception is
     a naked ape self-named *Homo sapiens.*
     Desmond Morris (1928–) British zoologist and writer.
     The Naked Ape, Introduction

22   Man's the bad child of the universe.
     James Oppenheim
     Laughter

23   The essence of being human is that one does not seek perfection.
     George Orwell (1903–50) British novelist.
     Shooting an Elephant, 'Reflections on Gandhi'

24   Man, as he is, is not a genuine article. He is an imitation of something, and
     a very bad imitation.
     P. D. Ouspensky (1878–1947) Russian-born occultist.
     The Psychology of Man's Possible Evolution, Ch. 2

25   The proper study of Mankind is Man.
     Alexander Pope (1688–1744) English poet.
     An Essay on Man, Epistle II

26   Man is Heaven's masterpiece.
     Francis Quarles (1592–1644) English writer.
     Emblems, Bk. II

27   Man is not a solitary animal, and so long as social life survives, self-realiza-
     tion cannot be the supreme principle of ethics.
     Bertrand Russell (1872–1970) British philosopher.
     History of Western Philosophy, 'Romanticism'

28   The mass of mankind is divided into two classes, the Sancho Panzas who

have a sense for reality, but no ideals, and the Don Quixotes with a sense for ideals, but mad.
George Santayana (1863–1952) Spanish-born US philosopher, poet, and critic.
Interpretations of Poetry and Religion, Preface

29 I love mankind – it's people I can't stand.
Charles M. Schultz (1922–) US cartoonist.
Go Fly a Kite, Charlie Brown

30 Because he is the highest vertebrate he can do what no other vertebrate can do: when, out of whatever desire and knowledge may be his, he makes a choice, he can say 'I will.' . . . And knowing how and why he says 'I will', he comes to his own as a philosopher.
Homer W. Smith (1895–1962)
From Fish to Philosopher, Ch. 13

31 The fish in the water is silent, the animal on the earth is noisy, the bird in the air is singing.
But Man has in him the silence of the sea, the noise of the earth and the music of the air.
Rabindranath Tagore (1861–1941) Indian poet and philosopher.
Stray Birds, 43

32 Man is a museum of diseases, a home of impurities; he comes today and is gone tomorrow; he begins as dirt and departs as stench.
Mark Twain (Samuel L. Clemens; 1835–1919) US writer.

33 The noblest work of God? Man. Who found it out? Man.
Mark Twain
Autobiography

34 We should expect the best and the worst from mankind, as from the weather.
Marquis de Luc de Clapiers Vauvenargues (1715–47) French moralist.
Reflections and Maxims, 102

35 We're all of us guinea pigs in the laboratory of God. Humanity is just a work in progress).
Tennessee Williams (1911–83) US dramatist.
Camino Real, 12

MASTURBATION

1 Don't knock it, it's sex with someone you love.
Woody Allen (Allen Stewart Konigsberg; 1935–) US film actor and director.

2 It is called in our schools 'beastliness' and this is about the best name for it

. . . should it become a habit it quickly destroys both health and spirits; he becomes feeble in body and mind, and often ends in a lunatic asylum.
Robert Baden-Powell (1857–1941) British general, founder of the Boy Scouts.
Scouting for Boys

3   And Onan knew that the seed should not be his; and it came to pass, when he went in unto his brother's wife that he spilled it on the ground, lest that he should give seed to his brother.
Bible: Genesis
38:9
Hence the term *Onanism* for masturbation or, sometimes, coitus interruptus

4   Because he spills his seed on the ground.
Dorothy Parker (1893–1967) US writer and wit.
Attrib.
Explaining why she called her canary 'Onan', see Genesis 38:9

5   One orgasm in the bush is worth two in the hand.
Robert Reisner
Graffiti, 'Masturbation'

6   Masturbation: the primary sexual activity of mankind. In the nineteenth century it was a disease; in the twentieth it's a cure.
Thomas Szasz (1920–) US psychiatrist and writer.
The Second Sin

MEASLES

1   A Chicago Papa is so Mean he Wont let his Little Baby have More than One Measle at a time.
Eugene Field (1850–95) US poet and journalist.
Nonsense for Old and Young, 'A Mean Man'

2   Love is like the measles, we all have to go through it.
Jerome K. Jerome (1859–1927) British humorous writer.
Idle Thoughts of an Idle Fellow, 'On Being in Love'

3   They say love's like the measles – all the worse when it comes late in life.
Douglas Jerrold (1803–57) British dramatist.
Wit and Opinions of Douglas Jerrold, a Philanthropist

MEDICAL ESTABLISHMENT

1   The medical establishment has become a major threat to health.
Ivan Illich (1926–) Austrian sociologist.
Medical Nemesis

MEDICAL ETHICS

1 I will maintain the honour and noble tradition of the medical profession. A
  clinician shall behave towards his colleagues as he would have them behave
  towards him. A clinician shall deal honestly with patients and colleagues and
  strive to expose those physicians who engage in fraud and deception.
  Geneva code of ethics for the medical profession

2 Ethics and Science need to shake hands.
  Richard Clarke Cabot (1868–1939)
  The Meaning of Right and Wrong, Introduction

3 I have noticed a tendency on the part of an occasional elderly and distinguished man to think that the rules of medical ethics were meant for young
  fellows just starting out, but not for him.
  J. Chalmers Da Costa (1863–1933)
  The Trials and Triumphs of the Surgeon, Ch. 1

4 Life is short, the art long, opportunity fleeting, experience treacherous, judgment difficult. The physician must be ready, not only to do his duty himself,
  but also to secure the co-operation of the patient, of the attendants and of
  externals.
  Hippocrates (c. 460 BC–c. 357 BC) Greek physician.
  Aphorisms, I, 1
  Usually quoted in Latin as *Ars longa, vita brevis*

5 I swear by Apollo the physician, by Asclepius, by Health, by Panacea and by
  all the gods and goddesses, making them my witnesses, that I will carry out,
  according to my ability and judgment, this oath and this indenture. To hold
  my teacher in this art equal to my own parents; to make him partner in my
  livelihood; when he is in need of money to share mine with him; to consider
  his family as my own brothers and to teach them this art, if they want to
  learn it, without fee or indenture; to impart precept, oral instruction, and all
  other instruction to my own sons, the sons of my teacher, and to indentured
  pupils who have taken the physician's oath, but to nobody else. I will use
  treatment to help the sick according to my ability and judgment, but never
  with a view to injury and wrong-doing. Neither will I administer a poison to
  anybody when asked to do so, nor will I suggest such a course. Similarly, I
  will not give a woman a pessary to cause abortion. But I will keep pure and
  holy both in my life and my art. I will not use the knife, not even, verily,
  on sufferers from stone but I will give place to such as are craftsmen therein.
  Into whatsoever houses I enter, I will enter to help the sick, and I will abstain from all intentional wrong-doing and harm, especially from abusing the
  bodies of man or woman, bond or free. And whatsoever I shall see or hear in
  the course of my profession, as well as outside my profession in my intercourse with men, if it be what should not be published abroad, I will never
  divulge holding such things to be holy secret. Now if I carry out this oath,
  and break it not, may I gain for ever reputation among all men for my life

and for my art; but if I transgress it and forswear myself, may the opposite befall me.
Hippocrates (c. 460 BC–c. 357 BC) Greek physician.
The Hippocratic Oath

MEDICAL FEES

1   If you are too smart to pay the doctor, you had better be too smart to get ill.
African (Transvaal) proverb

2   Exploratory operation: a remunerative reconnaissance.
Anonymous

3   You give medicine to a sick man; the sick man hands you gold in return.
You cure his disease, he cures yours.
Anonymous

4   Three shapes a doctor wears. At first we hail
The angel; then the god, if he prevail.
Last, when the cure complete, he asks his fee.
A hideous demon he appears to be.
Anonymous
Doctor and Patient

5   Physicians of the utmost fame,
Were called at once; but when they came
They answered, as they took their fees,
'There is no Cure for this Disease.'
Hilaire Belloc (1870–1953) French-born British poet.
Bartlett's Unfamiliar Quotations (Leonard Louis Levinson)

6   Private practice and marriage – those twin extinguishers of science.
Paul Broca (1824–80)
Letter, 10 Apr 1851

7   No one should approach the temple of science with the soul of a money changer.
Sir Thomas Browne (1605–82) English physician and writer.

8   But modern quacks have lost the art,
And reach of life the sacred seat;
They know not how its pulses beat,
Yet take their fee and write their bill,
In barb'rous prose resolved to kill.
Anna Chamber (d. 1777)
Poems, Printed at Strawberry Hill

9   A fashionable surgeon like a pelican can be recognized by the size of his bill.
J. Chalmers Da Costa (1863–1933)
The Trials and Triumphs of the Surgeon, Ch. 1

10   'Is there no hope?' the sick man said,
The silent doctor shook his head,
And took his leave with signs of sorrow,
Despairing of his fee tomorrow.
John Gay (1685–1732) English poet and dramatist.

11   I used to wonder why people should be so fond of the company of their physician, till I recollected that he is the only person with whom one dares to talk continually of oneself, without interruption, contradiction or censure; I suppose that delightful immunity doubles their fees.
Hannah More (1745–1833) English writer.
Letter to Horace Walpole, 27 July 1789

12   One must not count upon all of his patients being willing to steal in order to pay doctor's bills.
Robert Tuttle Morris (1857–1945)
Doctors versus Folks, Ch. 3

13   The patient suffered from chronic remunerative appendicitis.
Delbert H. Nickson (1890–1951)

14   A hospital should also have a recovery room adjoining the cashier's office.
Francis O'Walsh
Bartlett's Unfamiliar Quotations (Leonard Louis Levinson)

15   The doctor demands his fees whether he has killed the illness or the patient.
Polish proverb

16   God heals, and the doctor takes the fee.
Proverb

17   Sickness soaks the purse.
Proverb

18   They, on the whole, desire to cure the sick; and, – if they are good doctors, and the choice were fairly put to them, – would rather cure their patient and lose their fee, than kill him, and get it.
John Ruskin (1819–1900) British art critic and writer.
The Crown of Wild Olive

19   Our doctor would never really operate unless it was necessary. He was just that way. If he didn't need the money, he wouldn't lay a hand on you.
Herb Shriner

20   Wonderful is the skill of a physician; for a rich man he prescribeth various admixtures and compounds, by which the patient is rought to health in many days at an expense of fifty pounds; while for a poor man for the same disease

he giveth a more common name, and prescribeth a dose of oil, which
worketh a cure in a single night charging fourpence therefor.
James Townley (1714–78)

21 Ah well, I suppose I shall have to die beyond my means.
Oscar Wilde (1856–1900) Irish-born British writer and wit.
On being told the cost of an operation

MEDICAL STUDENTS

1 Of all the lessons which a young man entering upon the profession of medicine needs to learn, this is perhaps the first – that he should resist the fascination of doctrines and hypotheses till he has won the privilege of such
studies by honest labor and faithful pursuit of real and useful knowledge.
William Beaumont (1785–1853) US physician.
Notebook

2 The education of the doctor which goes on after he has his degree is, after
all, the most important part of his education.
John Shaw Billings (1838–1913)
Boston Medical and Surgical Journal, 131:140, 1894

3 Can there be a better preparatory school for the physician than the study of
the natural sciences? I think not!
Theodor Billroth (1829–94) Prussian-born surgeon.
The Medical Sciences in the German Universities, Pt. II, Ch. 2

4 My students are dismayed when I say to them, 'Half of what you are taught
as medical students will in ten years have been shown to be wrong, and the
trouble is, none of your teachers knows which half.'
C. Sidney Burwell (1893–1967)
British Medical Journal, 2:113, 1956 (G.W. Pickering)

5 The great doctors all got their education off dirt pavements and poverty–not
marble floors and foundations.
Martin H. Fischer (1879–1962)
Fischerisms (Howard Fabing and Ray Marr)

6 The medical student is likely to be one son of the family too weak to labour
on the farm, too indolent to do any exercise, too stupid for the bar and too
immoral for the pulpit.
Daniel Coit Gilman (1831–1908)
Attrib.

7 The most essential part of a student's instruction is obtained, as I believe, not
in the lecture room, but at the bedside.
Oliver Wendell Holmes (1809–94) US writer and physician.
Medical Essays, 'Scholastic and Bedside Teaching'

8 In teaching the medical student the primary requisite is to keep him awake.
Chevalier Jackson (1865–1958)
The Life of Chevalier Jackson, Ch. 16

9 His mind must be strong indeed, if, rising above juvenile credulity, it can
maintain a wise infidelity against the authority of his instructors, and the be-
witching delusions of their theories.
Thomas Jefferson (1743–1826) US statesman.
Letter to Dr. Caspar Wistar, 21 June 1807

10 There are two objects of medical education: To heal the sick, and to advance
the science.
Charles H. Mayo (1865–1939) US physician.
Collected Papers of the Mayo Clinic and Mayo Foundation, 18:1093, 1926

11 School yourself to demureness and patience. Learn to innure yourself to
drudgery in science. Learn, compare, collect the facts.
Ivan Pavlov (1849–1936) Russian physiologist.
Bequest to the Academic Youth of Soviet Russia, 27 Feb 1936

12 The first staggering fact about medical education is that after two and a half
years of being taught on the assumption that everyone is the same, the student has to find out for himself that everyone is different, which is really
what his experience has taught him since infancy. And the second staggering
fact about medical education is that after being taught for two and half years
not to trust any evidence except that based on the measurements of physical
science, the student has to find out for himself that all important decisions
are in reality made, almost at unconscious level, by that most perfect and
complex of computers the human brain, about which he has as yet learnt almost nothing, and will probably go on learning nothing to the end of his
course – this computer which can take in and analyse an incredible number
of data in an extremely short time. And the data are mostly not of the hard
crude type with which that simple fellow the scientist has to deal, but are of
a much more subtle, human, and interesting character, each tinted in its own
colours of personality and emotion. All this the student has to discover for
himself which his teachers strangely pretend to believe that the secrets of
medicine are revealed only to those whose biochemical background is beyond
reproach.
Sir Robert Platt (1900–)
British Medical Journal, 2:551, 1965

13 If you want to get out of medicine the fullest enjoyment, be students all your
lives.
David Riesman (1867–1940)

14 Take care not to fancy that you are physicians as soon as you have mastered
scientific facts; they only afford to your understandings an opportunity of

bringing forth fruit, and of elevating you to the high position of a man of
art.
Armand Trousseau (1801–67)
Clinical Medicine, Vol. I, Introduction

15 Medical education is not completed at the medical school: it is only begun.
William H. Welch (1850–1934)
Bulletin of the Harvard Medical School Association, 3:55, 1892

MEDICINE

1 If every man would mend a man, then all the world would be mended.
Anonymous

2 Medicine is a science which hath been, as we have said, more professed than
laboured, and yet more laboured than advanced; the labour having been, in
my judgment, rather in a circle than in progression.
Sir Francis Bacon (1561–1626) English philosopher, lawyer, and politician.
Advancement of Learning, Bk. II

3 The poets did well to conjoin Music and Medicine in Apollo: because the office of medicine is but to tune this curious harp of man's body and to reduce
it to harmony.
Sir Francis Bacon
The Advancement of Learning, Bk. II

4 The prime goal is to alleviate suffering, and not to prolong life. And if your
treatment does not alleviate suffering, but only prolongs life, that treatment
should be stopped.
Christian Barnard (1922–   ) South African surgeon.

5 With certain limited exceptions, the laws of physical science are positive and
absolute, both in their aggregate, and in their elements – in their sum, and
in their details; but the ascertainable laws of the science of life are approximative only, and not absolute.
Elisha Bartlett (1804–55)
Philosophy of Medical Science, Pt. II, Ch. 2

6 Physician, heal thyself.
Bible: Luke
4:23

7 Medicine . . . the only profession that labours incessantly to destroy the reason
for its own existence.
Sir James Bryce (1838–1922) British liberal politician, historian, and ambassa-
dor to the USA.
Address, 23 Mar 1914

8 Among the arts, medicine, on account of its eminent utility, must always
hold the highest place.
Henry Thomas Buckle (1821–62)
Miscellaneous and Posthumous Works, Vol. II

9 Nature, time and patience are the three great physicians.
Bulgarian proverb

10 My first article of belief is based on the observation, almost universally confirmed in present knowledge, that what happens in our bodies is directed toward a useful end.
Walter B. Cannon (1871–1945) US physiologist.
The Way of an Investigator, 'Some Working Principles'

11 The Art of Medicine is in need really of reasoning, . . . for this is a conjectural art. However, in many cases not only does conjecture fail, but experience as well.
Celsus (25 BC–50 AD) Roman encyclopedist.
De re medicina

12 Philosophy, like medicine, has plenty of drugs, few good remedies, and hardly
any specific cures.
Nicolas Chamfort (1741–94) French writer and wit.
Maximes et pensées

13 The whole imposing edifice of modern medicine is like the celebrated tower
of Pisa – slightly off balance.
Charles, Prince of Wales (1948–) Eldest son of Elizabeth II.

14 Medicine can only cure curable diseases, and then not always.
Chinese proverb

15 To a physician, each man, each woman, is an amplification of one organ.
Ralph Waldo Emerson (1803–82) US poet and essayist.
Bartlett's Unfamiliar Quotations (Leonard Louis Levinson)

16 In the hands of the discoverer medicine becomes a heroic art. . . . Wherever
life is dear he is a demigod.
Ralph Waldo Emerson
Uncollected Lectures, 'Resources'

17 Patience is the best medicine.
John Florio (1553–1625) English lexicographer and translator.
First Frutes

18 Study sickness while you are well.
Thomas Fuller (1654–1734) English physician and writer.
Gnomologia

19 Medicine absorbs the physician's whole being because it is concerned with the
    entire human organism.
    Johann Wolfgang von Goethe (1749–1832) German poet, dramatist and scientist.

20 Comedy is medicine.
    Trevor Griffiths (1935–)
    Comedians, I

21 Medicine is as old as the human race, as old as the necessity for the removal
    of disease.
    Heinrich Haeser (1811–84)
    Lehrbuch der Geschichte der Medizin, Erste Periode

22 Solving the mysteries of heaven has not given birth to as many abortive findings as has the quest into the mysteries of the human body. When you think
    of yourselves as scientists, I want you always to remember everything you
    learn from me will probably be regarded tomorrow as the naive confusions of
    a pack of medical aborigines. Despite all our toil and progress, the art of
    medicine still falls somewhere between trout casting and spook writing.
    Ben Hecht (1894–1964)
    Miracle of the Fifteen Murderers

23 Life is short, the art long, opportunity fleeting, experience treacherous, judgment difficult.
    Hippocrates (c. 460 BC–357 BC) Greek physician.
    Aphorisms, 1
    Usually quoted in Latin as *Ars longa, vita brevis*

24 It is so hard to get anything out of the dead hand of medical tradition!
    Oliver Wendell Holmes (1809–94) US writer and physician.
    Medical Essays, 'Currents and Counter-Currents in Medical Science'

25 The truth is, that medicine, professedly founded on observation, is as sensitive to outside influences, political, religious, philosophical, imaginative, as is
    the barometer to the changes of atmospheric density.
    Oliver Wendell Holmes
    Medical Essays, 'Currents and Counter-Currents in Medical Science'

26 The only sure foundations of medicine are, an intimate knowledge of the
    human body, and observation on the effects of medicinal substances on that.
    Thomas Jefferson (1743–1826) US statesman.
    Letter to Dr. Caspar Wistar, 21 June 1807

27 Common sense is in medicine the master workman.
    Peter Mere Latham (1789–1875) US poet and essayist.

28 Medicine is a strange mixture of speculation and action. We have to cultivate

a science and to exercise an art. The calls of science are upon our leisure and our choice; the calls of practice are of daily emergence and necessity.
Peter Mere Latham

29   When you buy a pill and buy peace with it you get conditioned to cheap solutions instead of deep ones.
Max Lerner (1902–   ) US author and journalist.
The Unfinished Country

30   Medicine is not a lucrative profession. It is a divine one.
John Coakley Lettsom (1744–1815)
Letter to a friend, 6 Sept 1791

31   Medicine makes people ill, mathematics makes them sad and theology makes them sinful.
Martin Luther (1483–1546) German Protestant reformer.

32   Medical practice is not knitting and weaving and the labor of the hands, but it must be inspired with soul and be filled with understanding and equipped with the gift of keen observation; these together with accurate scientific knowledge are the indispensable requisites for proficient medical practice.
Maimonides (Moses ben Maimon; 1135–1204) Spanish-born Jewish philosopher and physician.
Bulletin of the Institute of the History of Medicine, 3:555, 1935

33   All interest in disease and death is only another expression of interest in life.
Thomas Mann (1875–1955) German novelist.
The Magic Mountain, 6

34   Medicine is a conjectural art.
Jean Nicolas Corvisart des Marets (1755–1821)

35   Medicine may be defined as the art or the science of keeping a patient quiet with frivolous reasons for his illness and amusing him with remedies good or bad until nature kills him or cures him.
Gilles Ménage (1613–92)
Ménagiana, Pt. III

36   The aim of medicine is surely not to make men virtuous; it is to safeguard and rescue them from the consequences of their vices.
H. L. Mencken (1880–1956) US journalist and editor.
Prejudices, 'Types of Men: the Physician'

37   Medicine is for the patient. Medicine is the people. It is not for the profits.
George Merck (1894–1957)

38   The art of medicine is my discovery. I am called Help-Bringer throughout the world, and all the potency of herbs is known to me.
Ovid (Publius Ovidius Naso; 43 BC–17 AD) Roman poet.
Metamorphoses
Spoken by Apollo

39   The art of medicine is generally a question of time.
     Ovid
     Remedia Amoris

40   Medicine sometimes snatches away health, sometimes gives it.
     Ovid
     Tristia

41   Medicine is not only a science; it is also an art. It does not consist of com-
     pounding pills and plasters; it deals with the very processes of life, which
     must be understood before they may be guided.
     Paracelsus (c. 1493–1541) Swiss physician and alchemist.
     Die grosse Wundarznei

42   This basis of medicine is sympathy and the desire to help others, and what-
     ever is done with this end must be called medicine.
     Frank Payne (1840–1910)
     English Medicine in the Anglo-Saxon Times

43   Medicine is an art, and attends to the nature and constitution of the patient,
     and has principles of action and reason in each case.
     Plato (427 BC–347 BC) Greek philosopher.
     Gorgias

44   And this is what the physician has to do, and in this the art of medicine
     consists: for medicine may be regarded generally as the knowledge of the
     loves and desires of the body, and how to satisfy them or not; and the best
     physician is he who is able to separate fair love from foul, or to convert one
     into the other; and he who knows how to eradicate and how to implant love,
     whichever is required, and can reconcile the most hostile elements in the
     constitution and make them loving friends, is a skilful practitioner.
     Plato
     Symposium

45   Medicine for the dead is too late.
     Quintilian (Marcus Fabius Quintilianus; c. 35 AD–c. 96 AD) Roman rhetorician and
     teacher.

46   Truth in medicine is an unattainable goal, and the art as described in books
     is far beneath the knowledge of an experienced and thoughtful physician.
     Rhazes (Ar-Razi; c. 865–c. 928) Persian physician and philosopher.
     History of Medicine (Max Neuburger)

47   Medicine is a noble profession but a damn bad business.
     Humphrey Rolleston (1862–1944) British physician.
     Attrib.

48   Medicine is an occupation for slaves.
     Benjamin Rush (c. 1745–1813)
     Autobiography

49 It is our duty to remember at all times and anew that medicine is not only a science, but also the art of letting our own individuality interact with the individuality of the patient.
Albert Schweitzer (1875–1965) Franco-German, medical missionary, philosopher, and theologian.

50 By medicine life may be prolonged, yet death
Will seize the doctor too.
William Shakespeare (1564–1616) English dramatist and poet.
Cymbeline, V:5

51 Optimistic lies have such immense therapeutic value that a doctor who cannot tell them convincingly has mistaken his profession.
George Bernard Shaw (1856–1950) Irish dramatist and critic.
Misalliance, Preface

52 Medical science is as yet very imperfectly differentiated from common curemongering witchcraft.
George Bernard Shaw
The Doctor's Dilemma, 'Preface on Doctors'

53 . . . the department of witchcraft called medical science.
George Bernard Shaw
The Philanderer

54 Medicine can never abdicate the obligation to care for the patient and to teach patient care.
Maurice B. Strauss (1904–74)
Medicine, 43:19, 1964

55 Apollo was held the god of physic and sender of disease. Both were originally the same trade, and still continue.
Jonathan Swift (1667–1745) Anglo-Irish priest, poet, and satirist.
Thoughts on Various Subjects, Moral and Diverting

56 The art of medicine was to be properly learned only from its practice and its exercise.
Thomas Sydenham (1624–89)
Medical Observations, Dedicatory Epistle

57 Formerly when religion was strong and science weak, men mistook magic for medicine, now, when science is strong and religion weak, men mistake medicine for magic.
Thomas Szasz (1920–   ) US psychiatrist and writer.
The Second Sin

MEDICINES
See **DRUGS.**

MEDITATION

1   I neglect God and his angels for the noise of a fly, for the rattling of a
    coach, for the whining of a door.
    John Donne (1573–1631) English poet.
    Sermons, 80

2   Self-reflection is the school of wisdom.
    Baltasar Gracián (1601–58) Spanish writer and Jesuit.
    The Art of Worldly Wisdom, 69

3   If thou may not continually gather thyself together, do it some time at least
    once a day, morning or evening.
    Thomas à Kempis (1380–1471) German monk and writer.
    The Imitation of Christ, 1

4   Meditation is not a means to an end. It is both the means and the end.
    Krishnamurti
    The Second Penguin Krishnamurti Reader, Ch. 14

5   Nowhere can man find a quieter or more untroubled retreat than in his own
    soul.
    Marcus Aurelius (Marcus Aurelius Antoninus; 121–180) Roman emperor and Stoic
    philosopher.
    Meditations, 4

6   Self-knowledge is a dangerous thing, tending to make man shallow or insane.
    Karl Shapiro (1913–   ) US poet, critic, and editor.
    The Bourgeois Poet, 3

7   Explore thyself. Herein are demanded the eye and the nerve.
    Henry David Thoreau (1817–62) US writer.
    Walden, 'Conclusions'

MEMORY

1   Only stay quiet while my mind remembers
    The beauty of fire from the beauty of embers.
    John Masefield (1878–1967) British poet.
    On Growing Old

2   The young have aspirations that never come to pass, the old have reminis-
    cences of what never happened.
    Saki (Hector Hugh Munro; 1870–1916) British writer.
    Reginald at the Carlton

MEN

1   A sick man is as wayward as a child . . .
    Mary Russell Mitford (1787–1855) British writer.
    Julian, I:1

2   He is proud that he has the biggest brain of all the primates, but attempts to
    conceal the fact that he also has the biggest penis.
    Desmond Morris (1928–) British zoologist and writer.
    The Naked Ape, Introduction

MENTAL ILLNESS
See also **NEUROSIS, PSYCHIATRY, PSYCHOLOGY, SANITY, SCHIZ-
OPHRENIA.**

1   Lucid intervals and happy pauses.
    Sir Francis Bacon (1561–1626) English philosopher.
    The History of the Reign of King Henry VII

2   I cultivate my hysteria with joy and terror. Now I am always dizzy, and to-
    day, January 23, 1862, I experienced a singular premonition, I felt pass over
    me a breath of wind from the wings of madness.
    Charles Baudelaire (1821–67) French poet.
    Journaux intimes, 'Fusées', XVI

3   We all are born mad. Some remain so.
    Samuel Beckett (1906–) Irish novelist and dramatist.
    Waiting for Godot, II

4   'Mad' is a term we use to describe a man who is obsessed with one idea and
    nothing else.
    Ugo Betti (1892–1953) Italian dramatist.
    Struggle Till Dawn, 1

5   All of us are mad. If it weren't for the fact every one of us is slightly abnor-
    mal, there wouldn't be any point in giving each person a separate name.
    Ugo Betti
    The Fugitive, 2

6   All are lunatics, but he who can analyze his delusion is called a philosopher.
    Ambrose Bierce (1842–c. 1914) US writer and journalist.
    Epigrams

7   The wish to hurt, the momentary intoxication with pain, is the loophole
    through which the pervert climbs into the minds of ordinary men.
    Jacob Brownowski (1908–74) British mathematician and scientist.
    The Face of Violence, Ch. 5

8   The madman is not the man who has lost his reason. The madman is the
    man who has lost everything except his reason.
    G. K. Chesterton (1874–1936) British writer.
    Orthodoxy, Ch. 1

9   A mental stain can neither be blotted out by the passage of time nor washed
    away by any waters.
    Cicero (106 BC–43 BC) Roman orator and statesman.
    De Legibus, Bk. II

10 Diseases of the soul are more dangerous and more numerous than those of the
    body.
    Cicero
    Tusculanarum Disputationum, Bk III, Ch. 3

11 In a disordered mind, as in a disordered body, soundness of health is
    impossible.
    Cicero
    Tusculanarum Disputationum, Bk. III

12 Much Madness is divinest Sense–
    To a discerning Eye–
    Much Sense–the starkest Madness–
    Emily Dickinson (1830–86) US poet.
    Poems, 'Much Madness is Divinest Sense'

13 There is less harm to be suffered in being mad among madmen than in being
    sane all by oneself.
    Denis Diderot (1713–84) French writer and editor.
    Supplement to Bougainville's 'Voyage'

14 There is a pleasure sure
    In being mad which none but madmen know.
    John Dryden (1631–1700) English poet and dramatist.
    The Spanish Friar, 2

15 Where does one go from a world of insanity?
    Somewhere on the other side of despair.
    T. S. Eliot (1888–1965) US-born British poet and dramatist.
    The Family Reunion, II:2

16 Had there been a Lunatic Asylum in the suburbs of Jerusalem, Jesus Christ
    would infallibly have been shut up in it at the outset of his public career.
    Havelock Ellis (1859–1939) British psychologist.
    Impressions and Comments, 5 Jan 1922

17 The place where optimism most flourishes is the lunatic asylum.
    Havelock Ellis
    The Dance of Life, Ch. 3

18 Sanity is very rare: every man almost, and every woman, has a dash of
    madness.
    Ralph Waldo Emerson (1803–82) US poet and essayist.
    Journals

19 If you are physically sick, you can elicit the interest of a battery of physi-
    cians; but if you are mentally sick, you are lucky if the janitor comes around.
    Martin H. Fischer (1879–1962)
    Fischerisms (Howard Fabing and Ray Marr)

20 When a man lacks mental balance in pneumonia he is said to be delirious.
    When he lacks mental balance without the pneumonia, he is pronounced in-
    sane by all smart doctors.
    Martin H. Fischer
    Fischerisms (Howard Fabing and Ray Marr)

21 It is his reasonable conversation which mostly frightens us in a madman.
    Anatole France (Anatole François Thibault; 1844–1924) French writer.

22 Madness is part of all of us, all the time, and it comes and goes, waxes and
    wanes.
    Otto Friedrich

23 What is madness
    To those who only observe, is often wisdom
    To those to whom it happens.
    Christopher Fry (1907–) British dramatist.
    A Phoenix Too Frequent

24 I saw the best minds of my generation destroyed by madness, starving hysteri-
    cal naked.
    Allen Ginsberg (1926–) US poet.
    Howl

25 The world is so full of simpletons and madmen, that one need not seek them
    in a madhouse.
    Johann Wolfgang von Goethe (1749–1832) German poet, dramatist, and
    scientist.
    Conversations with Goethe, 17 Mar 1830 (Johann Peter Eckermann)

26 Ordinarily he is insane, but he has lucid moments when he is only stupid.
    Heinrich Heine (1797–1856) German poet and writer.
    Comment about Savoye, appointed ambassador to Frankfurt by Lamartine,
    1848

27 Insanity is often the logic of an accurate mind overtaxed.
    Oliver Wendell Holmes (1809–94) US writer and physician.

28 Every one is more or less mad on one point.
    Rudyard Kipling (1865–1936) Indian-born British writer and poet.
    Plain Tales from the Hills, 'On the Strength of a Likeness'

29 Madness need not be all breakdown. It may also be break-through. It is potential liberation and renewal as well as enslavement and existential death.
    R. D. Laing (1927–) British psychiatrist.
    The Politics of Experience, Ch. 16

30 Insanity is hereditary – you can get it from your children.
    Sam Levinson

31 The great proof of madness is the disproportion of one's designs to one's means.
    Napoleon I (Napoleon Bonaparte; 1769–1821) French emperor.
    Maxims

32 Insanity in individuals is something rare–but in groups, parties, nations, and epochs it is the rule.
    Friedrich Nietzsche (1844–1900) German philosopher.
    Beyond Good and Evil, Ch. 4

33 A sick mind cannot endure any harshness.
    Ovid (Publius Ovidius Naso; 43 BC–17 AD) Roman poet.
    Epistulae ex Ponto, Bk. I

34 All things can corrupt perverted minds.
    Ovid
    Tristia, Bk. II

35 The mind grows sicker than the body in contemplation of its suffering.
    Ovid
    Tristia, Bk. IV

36 Men are so necessarily mad, that not to be mad would amount to another form of madness.
    Blaise Pascal (1623–62) French philosopher and mathematician.
    Pensées, 414

37 His father's sister had bats in the belfry and was put away.
    Eden Phillpotts (1862–1960) British novelist and dramatist.
    Peacock House and Other Mysteries, 'My First Murder'

38 Those whom the Gods wish to destroy, they first drive mad.
    Proverb

39 One of the symptoms of approaching nervous breakdown is the belief that one's work is terribly important. If I were a medical man, I should prescribe a holiday to any patient who considered his work important.
    Bertrand Russell (1872–1970) British philosopher.
    The Autobiography of Bertrand Russell, Vol II: 1914–1944, Ch. 5

40 Sanity is madness put to good uses; waking life is a dream controlled.
    George Santayana (1863–1952) Spanish-born US philosopher, poet and critic.

41 Our occasional madness is less wonderful than our occasional sanity.
George Santayana
Interpretations of Poetry and Religion

42 A body seriously out of equilibrium, either with itself or with its environment, perishes outright. Not so a mind. Madness and suffering can set themselves no limit.
George Santayana
The Life of Reason: Reason in Common Sense, 2

43 Though this be madness, yet there is method in't.
William Shakespeare (1564–1616) English dramatist and poet.
Hamlet, II:2

44 I am but mad north-north-west. When the wind is southerly I know a hawk
from a handsaw.
William Shakespeare
Hamlet, II:2

45 MACBETH. Canst thou not minister to a mind diseas'd,
Pluck from the memory a rooted sorrow,
Raze out the written troubles of the brain,
And with some sweet oblivious antidote
Cleanse the stuff'd bosom of that perilous stuff
Which weighs upon the heart?
DOCTOR. Therein the patient
Must minister to himself.
MACBETH. Throw physic to the dogs,
I'll none of it!
William Shakespeare
Macbeth, V:3

46 We want a few mad people now. See where the sane ones have landed us!
George Bernard Shaw (1856–1950) Irish dramatist and critic.
Saint Joan

47 The madman thinks the rest of the world crazy.
Publilius Syrus (1st century BC) Roman dramatist.
Moral Sayings, 386

48 Whom Fortune wishes to destroy she first makes mad.
Publilius Syrus
Moral Sayings, 911

49 Pain of mind is worse than pain of body.
Publilius Syrus
Sententiae

50 We must remember that every 'mental' symptom is a veiled cry of anguish.

Against what? Against oppression, or what the patient experiences as oppression. The oppressed speak a million tongues . . . .
Thomas Szasz (1920–   ) US psychiatrist.

51   In the past, men created witches: now they create mental patients.
Thomas Szasz

52   When we remember that we are all mad, the mysteries disappear and life stands explained.
Mark Twain (Samuel L. Clemens; 1835–1910) US writer.

53   Men will always be mad and those who think they can cure them are the maddest of all.
Voltaire (François-Marie Arouet; 1694–1778) French writer and philosopher.
Letter, 1762

54   What is madness? To have erroneous perceptions and to reason correctly from them.
Voltaire
Philosophical Dictionary, 'Madness'

MIDDLE AGE
See also **AGE, ADOLESCENCE, OLD AGE, YOUTH.**

1   Years ago we discovered the exact point the dead centre of middle age. It occurs when you are too young to take up golf and too old to rush up to the net.
Franklin P. Adams (1881–1960) US journalist and humorist.
Nods and Becks

2   You've reached middle age when all you exercise is caution.
Anonymous

3   When you are forty, half of you belongs to the past . . . And when you are seventy, nearly all of you.
Jean Anouilh (1910–87) French dramatist.

4   A man of forty today has nothing to worry him but falling hair, inability to button the top button, failing vision, shortness of breath, a tendency of the collar to shut off all breathing, trembling of the kidneys to what ever tune the orchestra is playing, and a general sense of giddiness when the matter of rent is brought up. Forty is Life's Golden Age.
Robert Benchley (1889–1945) US humorist.
Bartlett's Unfamiliar Quotations (Leonard Louis Levinson)

5   A lady of a 'certain age', which means
Certainly aged.
George Gordon, Lord Byron (1788–1824) British poet.
Don Juan, VI

6   This day I am thirty years old. Let me now bid a cheerful adieu to my youth. My young days are now surely over, and why should I regret them? Were I never to grow old I might be always here, and might never bid farewell to sin and sorrow.
    Janet Colquhoun (1781–1846)
    Diary entry, 17 Apr 1811

7   When a middle-aged man says in a moment of weariness that he is half dead, he is telling the literal truth.
    Elmer Davis (1890–1958) US journalist.
    By *Elmer Davis*, 'On not being Dead, as Reported'

8   Middle age is youth without its levity,
    And age without decay.
    Daniel Defoe (1660–1731) English journalist and writer.

9   Middle age is when your age starts to show around the middle.
    Bob Hope (1904–   ) British-born US comedian.
    Attrib.

10 I think middle age is the best time, if we can escape the fatty degeneration of the conscience which often sets in at about fifty.
    W. R. Inge (1860–1954) British churchman and writer.
    Observer, 8 June 1930

11 The British loathe the middle-aged and I await rediscovery at 65, when one is too old to be in anyone's way.
    Roy Strong (1935–   ) British art critic.
    Remark, Jan 1988

12 In a man's middle years there is scarcely a part of the body he would hesitate to turn over to the proper authorities.
    E. B. White (1899–   ) US journalist and humorist.
    The Second Tree from the Corner, 'A Weekend with the Angels'

MIND

1   A great many open minds should be closed for repairs.
    Toledo Blade

2   Minds like bodies, will often fall into a pimpled, ill-conditioned state from mere excess of comfort.
    Charles Dickens (1812–70) British novelist.
    Barnaby Rudge, Ch. 7

3   We should take care not to make the intellect our god; it has, of course, powerful muscles, but no personality.
    Albert Einstein (1879–1955) German-born US physicist.
    Out of My Later Life, 51

4   The mind is an iceberg it floats with only 1/7 of its bulk above water.
    Sigmund Freud (1856–1939) Austrian psychoanalyst.
    Bartlett's Unfamiliar Quotations (Leonard Louis Levinson)

5   The conscious mind may be compared to a fountain playing in the sun and
    falling back into the great subterranean pool of subconscious from which it
    rises.
    Sigmund Freud
    Bartlett's Unfamiliar Quotations (Leonard Louis Levinson)

6   My life and work has been aimed at one goal only: to infer or guess how the
    mental apparatus is constructed and what forces interplay and counteract in
    it.
    Sigmund Freud
    Life and Work of Sigmund Freud (E. Jones)

7   The remarkable thing about the human mind is its range of limitations.
    Celia Green
    The Decline and Fall of Science, 'Aphorisms'

8   Little minds are interested in the extraordinary; great minds in the
    commonplace.
    Elbert Hubbard (1856–1915) US writer and editor.
    Roycroft Dictionary and Book of Epigrams

9   The natural course of the human mind is certainly from credulity to
    scepticism.
    Thomas Jefferson (1743–1826) US statesman.
    Letter to Dr. Caspar Wistar, 21 June 1807

10 The pendulum of the mind oscillates between sense and nonsense, not be-
    tween right and wrong.
    C. G. Jung (1865–1961) Swiss psychologist.
    Memories, Dreams, Reflections, Ch. 5

11 The highest function of *mind* is its function of messenger.
    D. H. Lawrence (1885–1930) British writer.
    Kangaroo, Ch. 16

12 The mind like a sick body can be healed and changed by medicine.
    Lucretius (c. 96 BC–55 BC) Roman philosopher and poet.
    On the Nature of Things, III

13 Mind is ever the ruler of the universe.
    Plato (429 BC–347 BC) Greek philosopher.
    Philebus

14 Happiness is beneficial for the body, but it is grief that develops the powers
    of the mind.
    Marcel Proust (1871–1922) French novelist.
    A la recherche du temps perdu: Le Temps retrouvé, Ch. 3

15   Once we are destined to live out our lives in the prison of our mind, our one
duty is to furnish it well.
Peter Ustinov (1921–   ) British actor, director, and writer.
Dear Me, Ch. 20

16   When people will not weed their own minds, they are apt to be overrun with
nettles.
Horace Walpole (1717–97) English writer.
Letter to Lady Ailesbury, 10 July 1779

17   The mind can also be an erogenous zone.
Raquel Welch (Raquel Tejada; 1940–   ) US film star.
Colombo's Hollywood (J. R. Colombo)

18   At 83 Shaw's mind was perhaps not quite as good as it used to be, but it was
still better than anyone else's.
Alexander Woollcott (1887–1943) US journalist.
While Rome Burns
Referring to George Bernard Shaw

MIND AND BODY

1   Disease is an experience of mortal mind. It is fear made manifest on the
body.
Mary Baker Eddy (1821–1910) US religious reader and scientist.
Science and Health, Ch. 14

2   If you start to think about your physical or moral condition, you usually find
that you are sick.
Johann Wolfang von Goethe (1749–1832) German poet and dramatist.
Sprüche in Prosa, Pt. I, Bk. II

3   We have rudiments of reverence for the human body, but we consider as
nothing the rape of the human mind.
Eric Hoffer (1902–   ) US writer.
Bartlett's Unfamiliar Quotations (Leonard Louis Levinson)

4   What we think and feel and are is to a great extent determined by the state
of our ductless glands and our viscera.
Aldous Huxley (1894–1964) British writer.
Music at Night, 'Meditation on El Greco'

5   The soul is subject to health and disease, just as is the body. The health and
disease of both . . . undoubtedly depend upon beliefs and customs, which are
peculiar to mankind. Wherefore I call senseless beliefs and degenerate customs
. . . diseases of humanity.
Maimonides (Moses ben Maimon; 1135–1204) Spanish-born Jewish philosopher
and physician.
Aphorisms according to Galen

6 The mind has great influence over the body, and maladies often have their
   origin there.
   Molière (Jean Baptiste Poquelin; 1622–73) French dramatist.
   Love's the Best Doctor, III

7 Our minds are lazier than our bodies.
   Duc François de la Rochefoucauld (1613–80) French writer.
   Bartlett's Unfamiliar Quotations (Leonard Louis Levinson)

8 Mind over matter.
   Virgil (Publius Vergilius Maro; 70 BC–19 BC) Roman poet.
   Aeneid, Bk. VI

9 Most of the time we think we're sick, it's all in the mind.
   Thomas Wolfe (1900–38) US novelist.
   Look Homeward, Angel, Pt. 1, Ch. 1

MISTAKES

1 For want of timely care
   Millions have died of medicable wounds.
   John Armstrong (1710–79) English physician and poet.
   Art of Preserving Health

2 The blunders of a doctor are felt not by himself but by others.
   Ar-Rumi (836–896)

3 The medical errors of one century constitute the popular faith of the next.
   Alonzo Clark (1807–87)

4 What we call experience is often a dreadful list of ghastly mistakes.
   J. Chalmers Da Costa (1863–1933)
   The Trials and Triumphs of the Surgeon, Ch. 1

5 Ignorance is preferable to error; and he is less remote from the truth who be-
   lieves nothing, than he who believes what is wrong.
   Thomas Jefferson (1743–1826) US statesman.
   Notes on the State of Virginia

6 Let them learn their art properly or cease to practise it. A mistake in other
   professions is tolerable, but this is full of danger if its practitioners are not
   perfect. It ravages like a hidden domestic plague.
   Marcellus Palingenius (16th century)
   The Zodiac of Life, Bk. IV, 'Leo'

7 Physicians' faults are covered with earth, and rich men's with money.
   Proverb

8   The physician can bury his mistakes, but the architect can only advise his
    client to plant vines.
    Frank Lloyd Wright (1869–1959) US architect.
    New York Times Magazine, 4 Oct 1953

N

NARCOTICS

1   Cocaine isn't habit-forming. I should know – I've been using it for years.
    Tallulah Bankhead (1903–68) US actress.
    Pentimento (Lillian Hellman), 'Theatre'

2   OPIATE. An unlocked door in the prison of
    Identity. It leads into the jail yard.
    Ambrose Bierce (1842–c. 1914) US writer and journalist.
    The Devil's Dictionary

3   I'll die young, but it's like kissing God.
    Lenny Bruce (1923–66) US comedian.
    The Routledge Dictionary of Quotations (Robert Andrews)

4   Opium is pleasing to Turks, on account of the agreeable delirium it produces.
    Edmund Burke (1729–97) British politician.
    On the Sublime and Beautiful, 'On Taste'

5   Laudanum gave me repose, not sleep; but you, I believe, know how divine
    this repose is, what a spot of enchantment, a green spot of fountain and
    flowers and trees in the very heart of a waste of sands.
    Samuel Taylor Coleridge (1772–1834) British poet.

6   Thou hast the keys of Paradise, oh, just, subtle, and mighty opium!
    Thomas De Quincey (1785–1859) British essayist and critic.
    Confessions of an English Opium-Eater, Pt. II

7   Opium gives and takes away. It defeats the steady habit of exertion; but it
    creates spasms of irregular exertion! It ruins the natural power of life; but it
    develops preternatural paroxysms of intermitting power.
    Thomas De Quincey
    Confessions of an English Opium-Eater, Pt. II

8   'For me,' said Sherlock Holmes, 'there still remains the cocaine bottle.'
    Sir Arthur Conan Doyle (1859–1930) British writer, creator of Sherlock
    Holmes.
    The Sign of Four, 'The Strange Story of Jonathan Small'

9   There is only one reason why men become addicted to drugs, they are weak
    men. Only strong men are cured, and they cure themselves.
    Martin H. Fischer (1879–1962)
    Fischerisms (Howard Fabing and Ray Marr)

10   There is no flying without wings.
     French proverb

11   Opium . . . the Creator himself seems to prescribe, for we often see the scarlet
     poppy growing in the cornfields, as if it were foreseen that whatever there is
     hunger to be fed there must also be pain to be soothed.
     Oliver Wendell Holmes (1809–94) US writer and physician.
     Medical Essays, 'Currents and Counter-Currents in Medical Science'

12   Science and art are only too often a superior kind of dope, possessing this ad-
     vantage over booze and morphia: that they can be indulged in with a good
     conscience and with the conviction that, in the process of indulging, one is
     leading the 'higher life'.
     Aldous Huxley (1894–1964) British writer.
     Ends and Means, 'Beliefs'

13   Along with many scientists he considered the discovery of psychedelics one of
     the three major scientific break-throughs of the twentieth century, the other
     two being the splitting of the atom and the manipulation of genetic
     structures.
     Laura Huxley
     Referring to Aldous Huxley
     This Timeless Moment

14   To tell the story of Coleridge without the opium is to tell the story of Ham-
     let without mentioning the Ghost.
     Sir Leslie Stephen (1832–1904) British critic.
     Hours in a Library, 'Coleridge'

NATURE

1   Oh, the powers of nature. She knows what we need, and the doctors know
    nothing.
    Benvenuto Cellini (1500–71) Florentine goldsmith and sculptor.
    Autobiography

2   Nature is better than a middling doctor.
    Chinese proverb

3   Nature can do more than physicians.
    Oliver Cromwell (1599–1658) English soldier and statesman.

4   Nature heals, under the auspices of the medical profession.
    Haven Emerson (1874–1957)
    Lecture

5 Whatever Nature has in store for mankind, unpleasant as it may be, men must accept, for ignorance is never better than knowledge.
   Enrico Fermi (1901–54) Italian physicist.
   Atoms in the Family (Laura Fermi)

6 Here's good advice for practice: go into partnership with nature; she does more than half the work and asks none of the fee.
   Martin H. Fischer (1879–1962)
   Fischerisms (Howard Fabing and Ray Marr)

7 In a large proportion of cases treated by physicians, the disease is cured by nature, not by them.
   Sir John Forbes (1787–1861)

8 We must turn to nature itself, to the observations of the body in health and disease to learn the truth.
   Hippocrates (c. 460 BC–c. 377 BC) Greek physician.
   Aphorisms

9 Man's chief goal in life is still to become and stay human, and defend his achievements against the encroachment of nature.
   Eric Hoffer (1902–   ) US writer and philosopher.
   The Temper of Our Time, 'The Return of Nature'

10 Nature is a benevolent old hypocrite; she cheats the sick and the dying with illusions better than any anodynes.
   Oliver Wendell Holmes (1809–94) US writer and physician.
   Medical Essays, 'The Young Practitioner'

11 Though you drive away Nature with a pitchfork she always returns.
   Horace (Quintus Horatius Flaccus; 65 BC–8 BC) Roman poet.
   Epistles, I

12 The whole of nature is a conjugation of the verb to eat, in the active and the passive.
   W. R. Inge (1860–1954) British writer and clergyman.
   Outspoken Essays

13 The art of healing comes from nature not from the physician. Therefore the physician must start from nature, with an open mind.
   Paracelsus (c. 1493–1541) Swiss physician and alchemist.
   Seven Defenses, Ch. 4

14 The physician is only the servant of nature, not her master. Therefore it behooves medicine to follow the will of nature.
   Paracelsus
   Three Books on the French Disease, Bk. III, Ch. 11

15 I watched what method Nature might take, with intention of subduing the symptom by treading in her footsteps.
Thomas Sydenham (1624–89)
Medical Observations, 5, Ch. 2

16 Nature has always had more power than education.
Voltaire (François Marie Arouet; 1694–1778) French writer and philosopher.
Vie de Molière

NERVOUS SYSTEM

1 When you suffer an attack of nerves you're being attacked by the nervous system. What chance has a man got against a system?
Russell Hoban (1925–) US writer and illustrator.
The Lion of Boaz-Jachin and Jachin-Boaz, Ch. 13

NEUROSIS
See also **MENTAL ILLNESS, PSYCHIATRY, PSYCHOLOGY, SANITY, SCHIZOPHRENIA.**

1 The psychotic person knows that two and two make five and is perfectly happy about it; the neurotic person knows that two and two make four, but is terribly worried about it.
Anonymous

2 A mistake which is commonly made about neurotics is to suppose that they are interesting. It is not interesting to be always unhappy, engrossed with oneself, malignant and ungrateful, and never quite in touch with reality.
Cyril Connolly (1903–74) British journalist and writer.
The Unquiet Grave, Pt. II

3 The true believer is in a high degree protected against the danger of certain neurotic afflictions; by accepting the universal neurosis he is spared the task of forming a personal neurosis.
Sigmund Freud (1856–1939) Austrian psychoanalyst.
The Future of an Illusion, Ch. 8

4 There are those who have tried to dismiss his story with a flourish of the Union Jack, a psycho-analytical catchword or a sneer; it should move our deepest admiration and pity. Like Shelley and like Baudelaire, it may be said of him that he suffered, in his own person, the neurotic ills of an entire generation.
Christopher Isherwood (1904–86) British writer.
Exhumations
Referring to T. E. Lawrence

5   Idleness begets ennui, ennui the hypochondriac, and that a diseased body. No
    laborious person was ever yet hysterical.
    Thomas Jefferson (1743–1826) US statesman.
    Letter to Martha Jefferson, 28 Mar 1787

6   Neurosis is always a substitute for legitimate suffering.
    C. G. Jung (1875–1961) Swiss psychologist.

7   This is, I think, very much the Age of Anxiety, the age of the neurosis, be-
    cause along with so much that weighs on our minds there is perhaps even
    more that grates on our nerves.
    Louis Kronenberger (1904–) US writer, critic, and editor.
    Company Manners, 'The Spirit of the Age'

8   Modern neurosis began with the discoveries of Copernicus. Science made man
    feel small by showing him that the earth was not the centre of the universe.
    Mary McCarthy (1912–) US novelist.
    On the Contrary, 'Tyranny of the Orgasm'

9   Neurotic means he is not as sensible as I am, and psychotic means he's even
    worse than my brother-in-law.
    Karl Menninger (1893–) US psychiatrist.

10 Freud is all nonsense; the secret of neurosis is to be found in the family battle
    of wills to see who can refuse longest to help with the dishes. The sink is the
    great symbol of the bloodiness of family life. All life is bad, but family life is
    worse.
    Julian Mitchell (1935–) British writer and dramatist.
    As Far as You Can Go, I, Ch. 1

11 Neurosis has an absolute genius for malingering. There is no illness which it
    cannot counterfeit perfectly. . . . If it is capable of deceiving the doctor, how
    should it fail to deceive the patient?
    Marcel Proust (1871–1922) French novelist.
    A la recherche du temps perdu: Le Côté de Guermantes

12 Everything great in the world comes from neurotics. They alone have founded
    our religions and composed our masterpieces.
    Marcel Proust
    A la recherche du temps perdu: Le Côté de Guermantes

13 The 'sensibility' claimed by neurotics is matched by their egotism; they can-
    not abide the flaunting by others of the sufferings to which they pay an ever
    increasing attention in themselves.
    Marcel Proust
    A la recherche du temps perdu: Le Côté de Guermantes

14 Work and love – these are the basics. Without them there is neurosis.
    Theodor Reik

15 Neurosis is the way of avoiding non-being by avoiding being.
Paul Tillich (1886–1965) German-born US Protestant theologian and
philosopher.
The Courage to Be

NURSING
See also **HOSPITALS**.

1 Too often a sister puts all her patients back to bed as a housewife puts all her
plates back in the plate-rack – to make a generally tidy appearance.
Richard Asher (1912–   )
British Medical Journal, 2:967, 1947

2 If th' Christyan Scientists had some science an' th' doctors more Christyanity,
it wudden't make anny diff'rence which ye called in – If ye had a good
nurse.
Finley Peter Dunne (1867–1936) US humorist and journalist.
Mr. Dooley's Opinions, 'Christian Science'

3 It's better to be sick than nurse the sick. Sickness is single trouble for the
sufferer: but nursing means vexation of the mind, and hard work for the
hands besides.
Euripides (484 BC–406 BC) Greek dramatist.
Hippolytus, 186

4 . . . a good nurse is of more importance than a physician.
Hannah Farnham Lee (1780–1865)
The Log-Cabin; or, the World Before You

5 The trained nurse has given nursing the human, or shall we say, the divine
touch, and made the hospital desirable for patients with serious ailments re-
gardless of their home advantages.
Charles H. Mayo (1865–1939) US physician.
Collected Papers of the Mayo Clinic and Mayo Foundation, 13:1242, 1921

6 No *man*, not even a doctor, ever gives any other definition of what a nurse
should be than this – 'devoted and obedient'. This definition would do just
as well for a porter. It might even do for a horse. It would not do for a
policeman.
Florence Nightingale (1820–1910) British nurse.
Notes on Nursing

7 The trained nurse has become one of the great blessings of humanity, taking
a place beside the physician and the priest, and not inferior to either in her
mission.
Sir William Osler (1849–1919) Canadian physician.
Aequanimitas, with Other Addresses, 'Nurse and Patient'

8 *Talk of the patience of Job*, said a Hospital nurse, *Job was never on night duty*.
   Stephen Paget (1855–1926)
   Confessio Medici, Ch. 6

9 That person alone is fit to nurse or to attend the bedside of a patient, who is
   cool-headed and pleasant in his demeanour, does not speak ill of any body, is
   strong and attentive to the requirements of the sick, and strictly and indefati-
   gably follows the instructions of the physician.
   Sushruta (5th century BC)
   Sushruta-Samhitá, 'Sutrasthánam', Ch. 34

O

OBESITY

1 Outside every fat man there is an even fatter man trying to close in.
Kingsley Amis (1922–) British writer.
One Fat Englishman, Ch. 3

2 An adult is one who has ceased to grow vertically but not horizontally.
Anonymous

3 A fat paunch never bred a subtle mind.
Anonymous

4 The one way to get thin is to re-establish a purpose in life.
Cyril Connolly (1903–74) British writer and critic.
The Unquiet Grave

5 Imprisoned in every fat man a thin one is wildly signalling to be let out.
Cyril Connolly
The Unquiet Grave

6 Obesity is a mental state, a disease brought on by boredom and disappointment.
Cyril Connolly
The Unquiet Grave

7 I'm fat but I'm thin inside. Has it ever struck you that there's a thin man inside every fat man, just as they say there's a statue inside every block of stone?
George Orwell (1903–50) British novelist.
Coming Up for Air

8 Enclosing every thin man, there's a fat man demanding elbow-room.
Evelyn Waugh (1903–66) British novelist.
Officers and Gentlemen, Interlude

9 She fitted into my biggest armchair as if it had been built round her by someone who knew they were wearing armchairs tight about the hips that season.
P. G. Wodehouse (1881–1975) British-born US humorous novelist.
My Man Jeeves, 'Jeeves and the Unbidden Guest'

OBSTETRICS
See also **BIRTH.**

1 There must be love

Without love you will be merely skilful.
Frédérick Leboyer (1918–   ) French obstetrician.
Entering the World (M. Odent)

OLD AGE

1   Everyone faces at all times two fateful possibilities: one is to grow older, the other not.
    Anonymous

2   Its a sign of age if you feel like the day after the night before and you haven't been anywhere.
    Anonymous

3   The principal objection to old age is that there's no future in it.
    Anonymous

4   You are getting old when the gleam in your eyes is from the sun hitting your bifocals.
    Anonymous

5   As men draw near the common goal
    Can anything be sadder
    Than he who, master of his soul,
    Is servant to his bladder?
    Anonymous
    The Speculum, Melbourne, 1938

6   Ageing seems to be the only available way to live a long time.
    Daniel-François-Esprit Auber (1782–1871) French composer.
    Dictionnaire encyclopédique (E. Guérard)

7   When men desire old age, what else do they desire but prolonged infirmity?
    St. Augustine (354–430) Bishop of Hippo in North Africa.
    Of the Catechizing of the Unlearned, XVI

8   To me, old age is always fifteen years older than I am.
    Bernard Baruch (1870–1965) US financier and presidential advisor.

9   An old man looks permanent, as if he had been born an old man.
    H. E. Bates (1905–74) British novelist.
    Death in Spring

10 Tidy the old into tall flats. Desolation at fourteen storeys becomes a view.
    Alan Bennett (1934–   ) British dramatist.
    Forty Years On

11 Tranquillity comes with years, and that horrid thing which Freud calls sex is expunged.
E. F. Benson (1867–1940) British novelist.
Mapp and Lucia

12 I smoke 10 to 15 cigars a day, at my age I have to hold on to something.
George Burns (1896–) US comedian.
Attrib.

13 I'll keep going till my face falls off.
Barbara Cartland (1902–) British romantic novelist.
The Observer, 'Sayings of the Week', 17 Aug 1975

14 Old age is the out-patient's department of purgatory.
Lord Cecil (1869–1956) British statesman.
The Cecils of Hatfield House (David Cecil)

15 Man fools himself. He prays for a long life, and he fears an old age.
Chinese proverb

16 We grow old more through indolence, than through age.
Christina of Sweden (1626–89) Swedish queen.
Maxims (1660–1680)

17 It is not by muscle, speed, or physical dexterity that great things are achieved, but by reflection, force of character, and judgement; in these qualities old age is usually not only not poorer, but is even richer.
Cicero (106 BC–43 BC) Roman orator and statesman.
On Old Age, VI

18 In 1716 he had a paralytic stroke which was followed by senile decay. The story is famous of the broken man, hobbling to gaze at Kneller's portrait which showed him in the full splendour of manhood and murmuring, 'That was once a man'.
T. Charles Edwards and Brian Richardson
Referring to John Churchill, First Duke of Marlborough
They Saw it Happen

19 All diseases run into one, old age.
Ralph Waldo Emerson (1803–82) US poet and essayist.
Journals

20 Forty is the old age of youth; fifty is the youth of old age.
French proverb

21 No skill or art is needed to grow old; the trick is to endure it.
Johann Wolfgang von Goethe (1749–1832) German poet, dramatist and scientist.

22 Old men are twice children.
Greek proverb

23 The first sign of his approaching end was when my old aunts, while undress-
    ing him, removed a toe with one of his socks.
    Graham Greene (1904–) British novelist.
    Travels with My Aunt

24 You will recognize, my boy, the first sign of old age: it is when you go out
    into the streets of London and realize for the first time how young the police-
    men look.
    Seymour Hicks (1871–1949) British actor-manager.
    They Were Singing (C. Pulling)

25 The misery of a child is interesting to a mother, the misery of a young man
    is interesting to a young woman, the misery of an old man is interesting to
    nobody.
    Victor Hugo (1802–85) French poet, novelist, and dramatist.
    Les Misérables, 'Saint Denis'

26 The ageing man of the middle twentieth century lives, not in the public
    world of atomic physics and conflicting ideologies, of welfare states and super-
    sonic speed, but in his strictly private universe of physical weakness and men-
    tal decay.
    Aldous Huxley (1894–1964) British writer.
    Themes and Variations, 'Variations on a Philosopher'

27 A medical revolution has extended the life of our elder citizens without pro-
    viding the dignity and security those later years deserve.
    John F. Kennedy (1917–63) US statesman.
    Acceptance speech, Democratic National Convention, Los Angeles, 15 July
    1960

28 Prolonged and costly illness in later years robs too many of our elder citizens
    of pride, purpose and savings.
    John F. Kennedy
    Message to Congress on the Nation's Health Needs, 27 Feb 1962

29 When you have loved as she has loved you grow old beautifully.
    W. Somerset Maugham (1874–1965) British writer and doctor.
    The Circle

30 What makes old age hard to bear is not the failing of one's faculties, mental
    and physical, but the burden of one's memories.
    W. Somerset Maugham
    Points of View, Ch. 1

31 Growing old is a bad habit which a busy man has no time to form.
    André Maurois (Emile Herzog; 1885–1967) French writer.
    The Ageing American

32   Old age puts more wrinkles in our minds than on our faces.
Michel de Montaigne (1533–92) French essayist.
Essays, Bk. III, Ch. 2, 'Of Repentance'

33   Old age is an island surrounded by death.
Juan Montalvo

34   Senescence begins
And middle age ends,
The day your descendants,
Outnumber your friends.
Ogden Nash (1902–71) US poet.

35   All would live long, but none would be old.
Proverb

36   As you get older you become more boring and better behaved.
Simon Raven (1927–   ) British writer.
The Observer 'Sayings Of the Week', 22 Aug 1976

37   If you want to be a dear old lady at seventy, you should start early, say about
seventeen.
Maude Royden (1876–1956)

38   Old age is a disease which we cannot cure.
Seneca (c. 4 BC–65 AD) Roman author and statesman.
Epistulae ad Lucilium

39   Doth not the appetite alter? A man loves the meat in his youth that he can-
not endure in his age.
William Shakespeare (1564–1616) English dramatist and poet.
Much Ado About Nothing, II:3

40   The denunciation of the young is a necessary part of the hygiene of older
people, and greatly assists the circulation of their blood.
Logan Pearsall Smith (1865–1946) US writer.
All Trivia, 'Last Words'

41   There are so few who can grow old with a good grace.
Sir Richard Steele (1672–1729) Irish-born English essayist and dramatist.
The Spectator, 263

42   Man can have only a certain number of teeth, hair and ideas; there comes a
time when he necessarily loses his teeth, hair and ideas.
Voltaire (François-Marie Arouet; 1694–1778) French writer and philosopher.
Philosophical Dictionary

43   An aged man is but a paltry thing
A tattered coat upon a stick, unless

Soul clap its hands and sing.
W. B. Yeats (1865–1939) Irish poet.
Sailing to Byzantium

44 Dying while young is a boon in old age.
Yiddish proverb

P

PAIN

1 Medicine would be the ideal profession if it did not involve giving pain.
Samuel Hopkins Adams (1871–1958) US politician.
The Health Master, Ch. 3

2 Man endures pain as an undeserved punishment; woman accepts it as a natural heritage.
Anonymous

3 There was a faith-healer of Deal,
Who said, 'Although pain isn't real,
If I sit on a pin
And it punctures my skin,
I dislike what I fancy I feel.'
Anonymous
Limerick

4 The greatest evil is physical pain.
St. Augustine (354–430) Bishop of Hippo in rth Africa
Soliloquies, I

5 There is no point in being overwhelmed by the appalling total of human suffering; such a total does not exist. Neither poverty nor pain is accumulable.
Jorge Luis Borges (1899–1986) Argentinian writer.
Other Inquisitions, 'A New Refutation of Time'

6 Pain – has an Element of Blank –
It cannot recollect
When it begun – or if there were
A time when it was not –.
Emily Dickinson (1830–86) US poet.
Poem

7 Pain and death are a part of life. To reject them is to reject life itself.
Havelock Ellis (1859–1939) British psychologist.
On Life and Sex: Essays of Love and Virtue, 2

8 Much of your pain is self-chosen.
It is the bitter potion by which the physician within you heals your sick self.
Kahlil Gibran (1888–1931) Lebanese mystic and poet.
The Prophet, 'On Pain'

9   Time heals old pain, while it creates new ones.
    Hebrew proverb

10 The art of life is the art of avoiding pain.
    Thomas Jefferson (1743–1826) US statesman.
    Letter to Maria Cosway, 12 Oct 1786

11 Pain is life – the sharper, the more evidence of life.
    Charles Lamb (1775–1834) English essayist.
    Letter to Bernard Barton, 9 Jan 1824

12 It would be a great thing to understand Pain in all its meanings.
    Peter Mere Latham (1789–1875) US poet and essayist.
    General Remarks on the Practice of Medicine, Ch. 14

13 The new-born child does not realize that his body is more a part of himself
    than surrounding objects, . . . and it is only by degrees, through pain, that he
    understands the fact of the body.
    W. Somerset Maugham (1874–1965) British writer and doctor.
    Of Human Bondage, Ch. 13

14 I knew that suffering did not ennoble; it degraded. It made men selfish,
    mean, petty and suspicious. It absorbed them in small things . . . it made
    them less than men; and I wrote ferociously that we learn resignation not by
    our own suffering, but by the suffering of others.
    W. Somerset Maugham
    The Summing Up

15 But pain is perfect miserie, the worst
    Of evils, and excessive, overturnes
    All patience.
    John Milton (1608–74) English poet.
    Paradise Lost, Bk. VI

16 We are more sensible of one little touch of a surgeon's lancet than of twenty
    wounds with a sword in the heat of fight.
    Michel de Montaigne (1533–92) French essayist and moralist.

17 An hour of pain is as long as a day of pleasure.
    Proverb

18 We must all die. But that I can save him from days of torture, that is what I
    feel as my great and ever new privilege. Pain is a more terrible lord of man-
    kind than even death himself.
    Albert Schweitzer (1875–1965) French Protestant theologian, philosopher, and
    physician.
    On the Edge of the Primeval Forest, Ch. 5

19 Remember that pain has this most excellent quality: if prolonged it cannot be severe, and if severe it cannot be prolonged.
Seneca (c. 4 BC–65 AD) Roman author and statesman.
Epistulae ad Lucilium, XCIV

20 Pain is the correlative of some species of wrong – some kind of divergence from that course of action which perfectly fills all requirements.
Herbert Spencer (1820–1903) British philosopher and supporter of Darwinism.
The Data of Ethics, Ch. 15

21 Nothing begins and nothing ends
That is not paid with moan;
For we are born in others' pain.
And perish in our own.
Francis Thompson (1859–1907) British poet and critic.
'Daisy'

22 *Miseris succurrere disco.*
I learn to relieve the suffering.
Virgil (Publius Vergilius Maro; 70 BC–19 BC) Roman poet.
Aeneid, I
Motto on the seal of the New Jersey College of Medicine

23 Pain with the thousand teeth.
Sir William Watson (1858–1935) British poet.
The Dream of Man

PATHOLOGY

1 Ugliness is a point of view: an ulcer is wonderful to a pathologist.
Austin O'Malley (1858–1932)

PATIENTS
See also **DOCTORS AND PATIENTS.**

1 It is not a case we are treating; it is a living, palpitating, alas, too often suffering fellow creature.
John Brown (1810–82)
Lancet, 1:464, 1904

2 Once in a while you will have a patient of sense, born with the gift of observation, from whom you may learn something.
Oliver Wendell Holmes (1809–94) US writer and physician.
Medical Essays, 'The Young Practitioner'

3   What I call a good patient is one who, having found a good physician, sticks
    to him till he dies.
    Oliver Wendell Holmes
    Medical Essays, 'The Young Practitioner'

4   Never believe what a patient tells you his doctor has said.
    Sir William Jenner (1815–98) English physician and pathologist.
    Attrib.

5   First, the patient, second the patient, third the patient, fourth the patient,
    fifth the patient, and then maybe comes science. We first do everything for
    the patient; science can wait, research can wait.
    Béla Schick (1877–1967) Austrian pediatrician.
    Aphorisms and Facetiae of Béla Schick (I. J. Wolf)

6   The patient has been so completely taken to pieces that nobody is able to
    look on him again as a whole being. He is no longer an individual man but
    a jumble of scientific data.
    Kenneth Walker
    The Circle of Life, I, Ch. 1

PLASTIC SURGERY

1   Before I applied the pressure bandages to prevent swelling, I took a final look
    at my work. The woman before me was no longer forty-five but a lovely per-
    son with the taut firm beauty of youth.
    Dr. Robert Alyn Franklyn
    Beauty Surgeon

2   Anybody who is anybody seems to be getting a lift – by plastic surgery these
    days. It's the new world wide craze that combines the satisfactions of psychoa-
    nalysis, massage, and a trip to the beauty salon.
    Eugenia Sheppard (20th century)
    New York Herald-Tribune, 24 Feb 1958

POLIO

1   The people – could you patent the sun?
    Jonas E. Salk (1914–) US virologist.
    Famous Men of Science (S. Bolton)
    On being asked who owned the patent on his polio vaccine

POST-MORTEM

1   In the post-mortem room we witness the final result of disease, the failure of
    the body to solve its problems, and there is an obvious limit to what one can

learn about normal business transactions from even a daily visit to the bank-ruptcy court.
W. Russell, Lord Brain
Canadian Medical Association Journal, 83:349, 1960

PREGNANCY
See also **BIRTH, OBSTETRICS.**

1   Hanging head downwards between cliffs of bone, was the baby, its arms all but clasped about its neck, its face aslant upon its arms, hair painted upon its skull, closed, secret eyes, a diver poised in albumen, ancient and epic, shot with delicate spasms, as old as a Pharaoh in its tomb.
    Enid Bagnold (1889–   ) British writer.
    The Door of Life, Ch. 2

2   The history of man for the nine months preceding his birth would, probably, be far more interesting and contain events of greater moment than all the three-score and ten years that follow it.
    Samuel Taylor Coleridge (1772–1834) British poet.
    Miscellanies, Aesthetic and Literary

3   In men nine out of ten abdominal tumours are malignant; in women nine out of ten abdominal swellings are the pregnant uterus.
    Rutherford Morison (1853–1939)
    The Practitioner, Oct 1965

PREVENTIVE MEDICINE

1   The skilful doctor treats those who are well but the inferior doctor treats those who are ill.
    Ch'in Yueh-jen (c. 225 BC)

2   There is only one ultimate and effectual preventive for the maladies to which flesh is heir, and that is death.
    Harvey Cushing (1869–1939) US surgeon.
    The Medical Career and Other Papers, 'Medicine at the Crossroads'

3   An apple a day keeps the doctor away.
    English proverb

4   A well chosen anthology is a complete dispensary of medicine for the more common mental disorders, and may be used as much for prevention as cure.
    Robert Graves (1895–1985) British poet and novelist.
    On English Poetry, Ch. 29

5   The prevention of disease today is one of the most important factors in the line of human endeavor.
    Charles H. Mayo (1865–1939) US surgeon.
    Collected Papers of the Mayo Clinic and Mayo Foundation, 5:17, 1913

6   The aim of medicine is to prevent disease and prolong life, the ideal of medicine is to eliminate the need of a physician.
William J. Mayo (1861–1939) US physician.
National Education Association: Proceedings and Addresses, 66:163, 1928

7   When meditating over a disease, I never think of finding a remedy for it, but, instead, a means of preventing it.
Louis Pasteur (1822–95) French scientist.
Address to the Fraternal Association of Former Students of the Ecole Centrale des Arts et Manufactures, Paris, 15 May 1884

8   Nicotinic acid cures pellagra, but a beefsteak prevents it.
Henry E. Sigerist (1891–1957)
Atlantic Monthly, June 1939

9   *Prevention* of disease must become the goal of every physician.
Henry E. Sigerist
Medicine and Human Welfare, Ch. 3

PRIVATE MEDICINE
See **MEDICAL FEES.**

PSYCHIATRY
See also **MENTAL ILLNESS, MIND, NEUROSIS, PSYCHOLOGY, SANITY, SCHIZOPHRENIA.**

1   Just because you're paranoid doesn't mean you're not being followed.
Anonymous

2   The new definition of psychiatry is the care of the id by the odd.
Anonymous

3   The psychiatrist is the obstetrician of the mind.
Anonymous

4   I have myself spent nine years in a' lunatic asylum and have never suffered from the obsession of wanting to kill myself; but I know that each conversation with a psychiatrist in the morning, made me want to hang myself because I knew I could not strangle him.
Antonin Artaud (1896–1948) French theatre producer, actor, and theorist.

5   To us he is no more a person
Now but a climate of opinion.
W. H. Auden (1907–73) British poet.
In Memory of Sigmund Freud

6   Of course, Behaviourism 'works'. So does torture. Give me a no-nonsense,

down-to-earth behaviourist, a few drugs, and simple electrical appliances, and in six months I will have him reciting the Athanasian creed in public.
W. H. Auden
A Certain World, 'Behaviourism'

7   In today's highly complex society it takes years of training in rationalization, accommodation and compromise to qualify for the good jobs with the really big payoffs you need to retain a first-rate psychiatrist in today's world.
Russell Baker (1925–) US journalist.
The New York Times, 21 Mar 1968

8   Psychiatrist: A man who asks you a lot of expensive questions your wife asks you for nothing.
Sam Bardell (1915–)

9   Psychoanalysts are not occupied with the minds of their patients; they do not believe in the mind but in a cerebral intestine.
Bernard Berenson (1865–1959) US art historian.
Conversations with Berenson (Umberto Morra)

10 No man is a hero to his wife's psychiatrist.
Dr. Eric Berne
Bartlett's Unfamiliar Quotations (Leonard Louis Levinson)

11 Self-contemplation is infallibly the symptom of disease.
Thomas Carlyle (1795–1881) Scottish historian and essayist.
Characteristics

12 Psychiatry's chief contribution to philosophy is the discovery that the toilet is the seat of the soul.
Alexander Chase (1926–) US journalist.
Perspectives

13 Psychoanalysis is confession without absolution.
G. K. Chesterton (1874–1936) British writer.

14 I can think of no better step to signalize the inauguration of the National Health service than that a person who so obviously needs psychiatric attention should be among the first of its patients.
Winston Churchill (1874–1965) British statesman.
Speech, July 1948
Referring to Aneurin Bevan

15 Psychoanalysis is spending 40 dollars an hour to squeal on your mother.
Mike Connolly
Bartlett's Unfamiliar Quotations (Leonard Louis Levinson)

16 It is sometimes best to slip over thoughts and not go to the bottom of them.
Marie de Sévigné (1626–96) French letter-writer.
Letter to her daughter

17   Or look at it this way. Psychoanalysis is a permanent fad.
      Peter de Vries (1906–   ) US writer.
      Forever Panting, opening words

18   He formulated his ideas in extravagant and exclusive forms, which have since
      got quietly modified—I doubt whether psychoanalysts would now maintain
      that dreams of overcoats, staircases, ships, rooms, tables, children, landscapes,
      machinery, airships, and hats commonly represent the genitals.
      Rosemary Dinnage
      Observer, 20 July 1980
      Referring to Sigmund Freud

19   The trouble with Freud is that he never played the Glasgow Empire Saturday
      night.
      Ken Dodd (1931–   ) British comedian.
      TV interview, 1965

20   The psychic development of the individual is a short repetition of the course
      of development of the race.
      Sigmund Freud (1856–1939) Austrian psychoanalyst.
      Leonardo da Vinci

21   No doubt fate would find it easier than I do to relieve you of your illness.
      But you will be able to convince yourself that much will be gained if we suc-
      ceed in transforming your hysterical misery into common unhappiness.
      Sigmund Freud

22   The poets and philosophers before me have discovered the unconscious; I
      have discovered the scientific method with which the unconscious can be
      studied.
      Sigmund Freud

23   A man should not strive to eliminate his complexes, but to get into accord
      with them: they are legitimately what directs his conduct in the world.
      Sigmund Freud

24   The examined life has always been pretty well confined to a privileged class.
      Edgar Z. Friedenberg (1921–   ) US sociologist.
      The Vanishing Adolescent, 'The Impact of the School'

25   The man who once cursed his fate, now, curses himself – and pays his
      psychoanalyst.
      John W. Gardner (1912–   ) US public official.
      No Easy Victories, 1

26   Anybody who goes to see a psychiatrist ought to have his head examined.
      Samuel Goldwyn (Samuel Goldfish; 1882–1974) Polish-born US film producer.

27   Freud is the father of psychoanalysis. It has no mother.
      Germaine Greer (1939–   ) Australian-born British writer and feminist.
      The Female Eunuch

28 Fortunately, analysis is not the only way to resolve inner conflicts. Life itself remains a very effective therapist.
Karen Horney (1885–   )

29 If a patient is poor he is committed to a public hospital as 'psychotic'; if he can afford the luxury of a private sanitarium, he is put there with the diagnosis of 'neurasthenia'; if he is wealthy enough to be isolated in his own home under constant watch of nurses and physicians he is simply an indisposed 'eccentric'.
Pierre Marie Félix Janet (1859–1947) French psychologist and neurologist.
La Force et la faiblesse psychologiques

30 It is indeed high time for the clergyman and the psychotherapist to join forces.
C. G. Jung (1875–1961) Swiss psychoanalyst.
Modern Man in Search of a Soul, Ch. 11

31 Psychoanalysis cannot be considered a method of education if by education we mean the topiary art of clipping a tree into a beautiful artificial shape. But those who have a higher conception of education will prize most the method of cultivating a tree so that it fulfils to perfection its own natural conditions of growth.
C. G. Jung

32 Show me a sane man and I will cure him for you.
C. G. Jung
The Observer, 19 July 1975

33 Freud and his three slaves, Inhibition, Complex and Libido.
Sophie Kerr (1880–1965)
The Saturday Evening Post, 9 Apr 1932

34 Psychoanalysis is the disease it purports to cure.
Karl Kraus (1874–1936) Austrian writer.

35 The relation between psychiatrists and other kinds of lunatics is more or less the relation of a convex folly to a concave one.
Karl Kraus

36 The mystic sees the ineffable, and the psycho-pathologist the unspeakable.
W. Somerset Maugham (1874–1965) British writer and doctor.
The Moon and Sixpence, Ch. 1

37 If the nineteenth century was the age of the editorial chair, ours is the century of the psychiatrist's couch.
Marshall McLuhan (1911–81) Canadian sociologist.
Understanding Media, Introduction

38 Considered in its entirety, psychoanalysis won't do. It is an end product, moreover, like a dinosaur or a zeppelin; no better theory can ever by erected

on its ruins, which will remain for ever one of the saddest and strangest of all landmarks in the history of twentieth century thought.
Peter Medawar (1915–87) British immunologist.
The Hope of Progress

39 They have a financial interest in being wrong; the more children they can disturb, the larger their adult clientele.
Geoffrey Robinson
Hedingham Harvest
Referring to psychiatrists

40 The care of the human mind is the most noble branch of medicine.
Aloysius Sieffert (fl. 1858)
Medical and Surgical Practitioner's Memorandum

41 One should only see a psychiatrist out of boredom.
Muriel Spark (1918–   ) British novelist.

42 A psychiatrist is a man who goes to the Folies-Bergère and looks at the audience.
Mervyn Stockwood (1913–   ) British churchman.
The Observer, 'Sayings of the Week', 15 Oct 1961

43 Psychiatrists classify a person as neurotic if he suffers from his problems in living, and a psychotic if he makes others suffer.
Thomas Szasz (1920–   ) US psychiatrist.
The Second Sin

44 Like all analysts Randolph is interested only in himself. In fact, I have often thought that the analyst should pay the patient for allowing himself to be used as a captive looking-glass.
Gore Vidal (1925–   ) US novelist.
Myra Breckinridge, Ch. 37

45 Men will always be mad and those who think they can cure them are the maddest of all.
Voltaire (François Marie Arouet; 1694–1778) French writer and philosopher.
Letter, 1762

46 A neurotic is the man who builds a castle in the air. A psychotic is the man who lives in it. And a psychiatrist is the man who collects the rent.
Lord Robert Webb-Johnstone (1879–   )
Collected Papers

47 The ideas of Freud were popularized by people who only imperfectly understood them, who were incapable of the great effort required to grasp them in their relationship to larger truths, and who therefore assigned to them a prominence out of all proportion to their true importance.
Alfred North Whitehead (1861–1947) British philosopher and mathematician.
Dialogues, Dialogue XXVIII (June 3, 1943)

48 He was meddling too much in my private life.
Tennessee Williams (1911–83) US dramatist.
Attrib.
Explaining why he had given up visiting his psychoanalyst

49 He is always called a nerve specialist because it sounds better, but everyone
knows he's a sort of janitor in a looney bin.
P. G. Wodehouse (1881–1975) British-born US humorous novelist.
The Inimitable Jeeves

50 Daughters go into analysis hating their fathers, and come out hating their
mothers. They never come out hating themselves.
Laurie Jo Wojcik

PSYCHOANALYSIS
See **PSYCHIATRY**.

PSYCHOLOGY
See also **MIND, PSYCHIATRY**.

1   An animal psychologist is a man who pulls habits out of rats.
Anonymous

2   It seems a pity that psychology should have destroyed all our knowledge of
human nature.
G. K. Chesterton (1874–1936) British essayist, novelist, and poet.
Observer, 9 Dec 1934

3   Every day, in every way, I am getting better and better.
Emile Coué (1857–1926) French psychologist and pharmacist.
My Method, Ch. 3
Formula for a cure by auto-suggestion used at his clinic in Nancy

4   Popular psychology is a mass of cant, of slush and of superstition worthy of
the most flourishing days of the medicine man.
John Dewey (1859–1952) US philosopher.
The Public and Its Problems, Ch. 5

5   Psychology has a long past, but only a short history.
Hermann Ebbinghaus (1850–1909) German psychologist.
Summary of Psychology

6   The psychic development of the individual is a short repetition of the course
of development of the race.
Sigmund Freud (1856–1939) Austrian psychoanalyst.
Leonardo da Vinci

7   The separation of psychology from the premises of biology is purely artificial,
    because the human psyche lives in indissoluble union with the body.
    C. G. Jung (1875–1961) Swiss psychoanalyst.
    Factors Determining Human Behaviour, 'Psychological Factors Determining
    Human Behaviour'

8   Psychology is as unnecessary as directions for using poison.
    Karl Kraus (1874–1936) Austrian writer.

9   Thousands of American women know far more about the subconscious than
    they do about sewing.
    H. L. Mencken (1880–1956) US journalist.
    Prejudices

10 Psychology which explains everything
    explains nothing,
    and we are still in doubt.
    Marianne Moore (1887–1972) US poet.
    Collected Poems, 'Marriage'

11 Idleness is the parent of all psychology.
    Friedrich Nietzsche (1844–1900) German philosopher.
    Twilight of the Idols, 'Maxims and Missiles'

12 I never saw a person's id
    I hope I never see one.
    But I can tell you if I did
    I'd clamp an ego as a lid
    Upon the id to keep it hid,
    Which is, I gather, what God did
    When he first saw a free one.
    Helen Harris Perlman (1905–)
    National Association of Social Workers News, 9:2, 1964

13 A large part of the popularity and persuasiveness of psychology comes from its
    being a sublimated spiritualism: a secular, ostensibly scientific way of affirming
    the primacy of 'spirit' over matter.
    Susan Sontag (1933–) US novelist and essayist.
    Illness as Metaphor, Ch. 7

14 I maintain that today many an inventor, many a diplomat, many a financier
    is a sounder philosopher than all those who practise the dull craft of experi-
    mental psychology.
    Oswald Spengler (1880–1936) German philosopher.
    Decline of the West

15 There is no psychology; there is only biography and autobiography.
    Thomas Szasz (1920–) US psychiatrist.
    The Second Sin, 'Psychology'

16 Man, by the very fact of being man, by possessing consciousness, is, in comparison with the ass or the crab, a diseased animal. Consciousness is a disease.
Miguel de Unamuno y Jugo (1864–1937) Spanish writer and philosopher.
The Tragic Sense of Life, 1

17 The object of psychology is to give us a totally different idea of the things we know best.
Paul Valéry (1871–1945) French writer.
Tel quel

Q

QUACKS

1 Quackery gives birth to nothing; gives death to all things.
  Thomas Carlyle (1795–1881) Scottish essayist and historian.
  Heroes and Hero-Worship

2 Quacks are the greatest liars in the world except their patients.
  Benjamin Franklin (1706–90) US scientist and statesman.

3 The practice of physic is jostled by quacks on the one side, and by science
  on the other.
  Peter Mere Latham (1789–1875) US poet and essayist.
  Collected Works, Vol. I, 'In Memoriam' (Sir Thomas Watson)

4 Man is a dupable animal. Quacks in medicine, quacks in religion, and quacks
  in politics know this, and act upon that knowledge.
  Robert Southey (1774–1843) British poet.
  The Doctor, Ch. 87

5 By quack I mean imposter not in opposition to but in common with
  physicians.
  Horace Walpole (1717–97) English writer.

R

REMEDIES
See also **CURES, DIAGNOSIS, HEALING, TREATMENT.**

1   Here lie I and my four daughters,
    Killed by drinking Cheltenham waters.
    Had we but stick to Epsom salts,
    We wouldn't have been in these here vaults.
    Cheltenham Waters

2   Here lies the body of Mary Ann Lowder,
    She burst while drinking a seidlitz powder.
    Called from the world to her heavenly rest,
    She should have waited till it effervesced.
    Epitaph

3   Surely every medicine is an innovation, and he that will not apply new reme-
    dies, must expect new evils.
    Sir Francis Bacon (1561–1626) English philosopher, lawyer, and politician.
    Essays, 'Of Innovations'

4   The remedy is worse than the disease.
    Sir Francis Bacon
    Essays, 'Of Seditions and Troubles'

5   Well, now, there's a remedy for everything except death.
    Miguel de Cervantes (1547–1616) Spanish novelist.
    Don Quixote, Pt. II, Ch. 10

6   When a lot of remedies are suggested for a disease, that means it can't be
    cured.
    Anton Chekhov (1860–1904) Russian dramatist.
    The Cherry Orchard, II

7   A single untried popular remedy often throws the scientific doctor into
    hysterics.
    Chinese proverb

8   If you are too fond of new remedies, first you will not cure your patients; sec-
    ondly, you will have no patients to cure.
    Sir Astley Paston Cooper (1768–1841)

9   Every day, in every way, I am getting better and better.
    Emile Coué (1857–1926) French psychologist and pharmacist.
    My Method, Ch. 3
    Formula for a cure by auto-suggestion used at his clinic in Nancy

10   Life as we find it is too hard for us; it entails too much pain, too many dis-
     appointments, impossible tasks. We cannot do without palliative remedies.
     Sigmund Freud (1856–1939) Austrian psychoanalyst.
     Civilization and Its Discontents

11   Extreme remedies are most appropriate for extreme diseases.
     Hippocrates (c. 460 BC–c. 377 BC) Greek physician.
     Aphorisms, I

12   To do nothing is also a good remedy.
     Hippocrates
     Aphorisms, I

13   Remedies, indeed, are our great analyzers of disease.
     Peter Mere Latham (1789–1875) US physician.
     General Remarks on the Practice of Medicine, Ch. 7

14   Most men die of their remedies, and not of their illnesses.
     Molière (Jean-Baptiste Poquelin; 1622–73) French dramatist.
     Le Malade imaginaire, III:3

15   Men worry over the great number of diseases; doctors worry over the small
     number of remedies.
     Pien Ch'iao (c. 225 BC)

16   As soon as he ceased to be mad he became merely stupid. There are maladies
     we must not seek to cure because they alone protect us from others that are
     more serious.
     Marcel Proust (1871–1922) French novelist.
     A la recherche du temps perdu: Le Côté de Guermantes

17   Tis a sharp remedy, but a sure one for all ills.
     Sir Walter Raleigh (c. 1552–1618) English explorer and writer.
     Attrib.
     Referring to the executioner's axe just before he was beheaded

18   Our remedies oft in ourselves do lie,
     Which we ascribe to heaven.
     William Shakespeare (1564–1616) English dramatist and poet.
     All's Well That Ends Well, I:1

19   Our body is a machine for living. It is organized for that, it is its nature. Let
     life go on in it unhindered and let it defend itself, it will do more than if
     you paralyse it by encumbering it with remedies.
     Leo Tolstoy (1828–1910) Russian writer.
     War and Peace, Bk. X, Ch. 29

20   Three remedies of the physicians of Myddfai: water, honey, and labour.
     Welsh proverb

RESEARCH
See also **MEDICINE, SCIENCE.**

1   We vivisect the nightingale
    To probe the secret of his note.
    T. B. Aldrich (1836–1907) US writer and editor.

2   CLINICIAN: learns less and less about more and more until he knows nothing about everything.
    RESEARCHER: learns more and more about less and less until he knows everything about nothing.
    Anonymous

3   Research demands involvement. It cannot be delegated very far.
    Anonymous

4   We must discover the laws on which our profession rests, and not invent them.
    Anonymous

5   Celsus . . . tells us that the experimental part of medicine was first discovered, and that afterwards men philosophized about it; and hunted for and assigned causes; and not by an inverse process that philosophy and the knowledge of causes led to the discovery and development of the experimental part.
    Sir Francis Bacon (1561–1626) English philosopher, lawyer, and politician.
    Novum Organum, 'Aphorisms', LXXIII

6   Man can learn nothing except by going from the known to the unknown.
    Claude Bernard (1813–78) French physiologist.
    An Introduction to the Study of Experimental Medicine, Ch. 2

7   A first-rate laboratory is one in which mediocre scientists can produce outstanding work.
    Patrick Maynard Stuart Blackett (1897–1974)
    Attrib.

8   Many a man who is brooding over alleged mighty discoveries reminds me of a hen sitting on billiard balls.
    J. Chalmers Da Costa (1863–1933)
    The Trials and Triumphs of the Surgeon, Ch. 1

9   I must begin with a good body of facts and not from a principle (in which I always suspect some fallacy) and then as much deduction as you please.
    Charles Darwin (1809–82) British life scientist.
    Letter to J. Fiske, 8 Dec 1874

10 But in science the credit goes to the man who convinces the world, not to the man to whom the idea first occurs.
    Sir Francis Darwin (1848–1925) British scientist.
    Eugenics Review, 6:1, 1914

11   Every great advance in science has issued from a new audacity of imagination.
     John Dewey (1859–1952) US philosopher and educationalist.
     The Quest for Certainty, Ch. 11

12   No amount of experimentation can ever prove me right; a single experiment
     can prove me wrong.
     Albert Einstein (1879–1955) German physicist.

13   With a microscope you see the surface of things. It magnifies them but does
     not show you reality. It makes things seem higher and wider. But do not sup-
     pose you are seeing things in themselves.
     Feng-shen Yin-Te (1771–1810)
     The Microscope

14   None of the great discoveries was made by a 'specialist' or a 'researcher'.
     Martin H. Fischer (1879–1962)
     Fischerisms (Howard Fabing and Ray Marr)

15   Don't despise empiric truth. Lots of things work in practice for which the
     laboratory has never found proof.
     Martin H. Fischer
     Fischerisms (Howard Fabing and Ray Marr)

16   All the world is a laboratory to the inquiring mind.
     Martin H. Fischer
     Fischerisms (Howard Fabing and Ray Marr)

17   Research has been called good business, a necessity, a gamble, a game. It is
     none of these – it's a state of mind.
     Martin H. Fischer
     Fischerisms (Howard Fabing and Ray Marr)

18   I have been trying to point out that in our lives chance may have an aston-
     ishing influence and, if I may offer advice to the young laboratory worker, it
     would be this – never to neglect an extraordinary appearance or happening.
     It may be – usually is, in fact – a false alarm that leads to nothing, but it
     may on the other hand be the clue provided by fate to lead you to some im-
     portant advance.
     Alexander Fleming (1881–1955) Scottish bacteriologist.
     Lecture at Harvard

19   One does not discover new lands without consenting to lose sight of the
     shore for a very long time.
     André Gide (1869–1951) French novelist.
     The Counterfeiters

20   The way to do research is to attack the facts at the point of greatest
     astonishment.
     Celia Green
     The Decline and Fall of Science, 'Aphorisms'

21 Most of the knowledge and much of the genius of the research worker lie behind his selection of what is worth observing. It is a crucial choice, often determining the success or failure of months of work, often differentiating the brilliant discoverer from the . . . plodder.
Alan Gregg (1890–1957)
The Furtherance of Medical Research

22 The foundation of the study of Medicine, as of all scientific inquiry, lies in the belief that every natural phenomenon, trifling as it may seem, has a fixed and invariable meaning.
Sir William Withey Gull (1816–90)
Published Writings, 'Study of Medicine'

23 The great tragedy of Science: the slaying of a beautiful hypothesis by an ugly fact.
Thomas Huxley (1825–95) British biologist.
'Biogenesis and Abigenesis'

24 If . . . an outbreak of cholera might be caused either by an infected water supply or by the blasphemies of an infidel mayor, medical research would be in confusion.
W. R. Inge (1860–1954) British writer and churchman.
Outspoken Essays, 'Confessio Fidei'

25 Thus men of more enlighten'd genius and more intrepid spirit must compose themselves to the risque of public censure, and the contempt of their jealous contemporaries, in order to lead ignorant and prejudic'd minds into more happy and successful methods.
John Jones (1729–91)
Introductory lecture to his course in surgery

26 It is a good morning exercise for a research scientist to discard a pet hypothesis every day before breakfast.
Konrad Lorenz (1903–89) Austrian zoologist and pioneer of ethology.
On Aggression, Ch. 2

27 The aim of research is the discovery of the equations which subsist between the elements of phenomena.
Ernst Mach (1838–1916) Austrian physicist and philosopher.
Popular Scientific Lectures

28 Yet had Fleming not possessed immense knowledge and an unremitting gift of observation he might not have observed the effect of the hyssop mould. 'Fortune', remarked Pasteur, 'favours the prepared mind.'
André Maurois (Emile Herzog; 1885–1967) French writer.
Life of Alexander Fleming

29 The human body is private property. We have to have a search warrant to look inside, and even then an investigator is confined to a few experimental

tappings here and there, some gropings on the party wall, a torch flashed rather hesitantly into some of the dark corners.
Jonathan Miller (1936–) British writer and doctor.
BBC TV programme, *The Body in Question*, 'Perishable Goods', 15 Feb 1979

30 GERONTE. It was very clearly explained, but there was just one thing which surprised me – that was the positions of the liver and the heart. It seemed to me that you got them the wrong way about, that the heart should be on the left side, and the liver on the right.
SGANARELLE. Yes, it used to be so but we have changed all that. Everything's quite different in medicine nowadays.
Molière (Jean-Baptiste Poquelin; 1622–73) French dramatist.
Le Médecin malgré lui, II:4

31 Experiment alone crowns the efforts of medicine, experiment limited only by the natural range of the powers of the human mind. Observation discloses in the animal organism numerous phenomena existing side by side, and interconnected now profoundly, now indirectly, or accidentally. Confronted with a multitude of different assumptions the mind must *guess* the real nature of this connection.
Ivan Pavlov (1849–1936) Russian physiologist.
Experimental Psychology and Other Essays, Pt. X

32 Experience is the mother of science.
Proverb

33 It is with medicine as with mathematics: we should occupy our minds only with what we continue to know; what we once knew is of little consequence.
Charles Augustin Sainte-Beuve (1804–69) French critic.

34 It is too bad that we cannot cut the patient in half in order to compare two regimens of treatment.
Béla Schick (1877–1967) Austrian pediatrician.
Aphorisms and Facetiae of Béla Schick, 'Early Years' (I.J. Wolfe)

35 When I look back upon the past, I can only dispel the sadness which falls upon me by gazing into that happy future when the infection will be banished. . . . The conviction that such a time must inevitably sooner or later arrive will cheer my dying hour.
Ignaz Semmelweis (1818–65)
Etiology, Foreword
Semmelweis had discovered that it was the physicians who spread childbirth fever amongst patients.

36 We must also keep in mind that discoveries are usually not made by one man alone, but that many brains and many hands are needed before a discovery is made for which one man receives the credit.
Henry E. Sigerist (1891–1957)
A History of Medicine, Vol. I, Introduction

37   Research is fundamentally a state of mind involving continual reexamination
     of the doctrines and axioms upon which current thought and action are
     based. It is, therefore, critical of existing practices.
     Theobald Smith (1859–1934)
     American Journal of Medical Science, 178:741, 1929

38   We do not know the mode of action of almost all remedies. Why therefore
     fear to confess our ignorance? In truth, it seems that the words 'I do not
     know' stick in every physician's throat.
     Armand Trousseau (1801–67)
     Bulletin de l'académie impériale de médecine, 25:733, 1860

39   The outcome of any serious research can only be to make two questions grow
     where only one grew before.
     Thorsten Veblen (1857–1929) US social scientist.
     The Place of Science in Modern Civilization

40   It requires a very unusual mind to undertake the analysis of the obvious.
     A. N. Whitehead (1861–1947) British mathematician and philosopher.
     Science and the Modern World

S

SANITY

1 Outside, among your fellows, among strangers, you must preserve appearances, a hundred things you cannot do, but inside, the terrible freedom!
Ralph Waldo Emerson (1803–82) US poet and essayist.

2 Sanity is very rare; every man almost, and every woman, has a dash of madness.
Ralph Waldo Emerson

3 Who, then, is sane?.
Horace (65 BC–8 BC) Roman poet.

4 Sanity is a madness put to good uses; waking life is a dream controlled.
George Santayana (1863–1952) Spanish-born US philosopher, poet, and critic.
Interpretations of Poetry and Religion, Ch. 10

5 An asylum for the sane would be empty in America.
George Bernard Shaw (1856–1950) Irish dramatist and critic.

6 Every man has a sane spot somewhere.
Robert Louis Stevenson (1850–94) Scottish writer.
Bartlett's Unfamiliar Quotations (Leonard Louis Levinson)

7 The way it is now, the asylums can hold the sane people, but if we tried to shut up the insane we should run out of building materials.
Mark Twain (Samuel L. Clemens; 1835–1910) US writer.
Bartlett's Unfamiliar Quotations (Leonard Louis Levinson)

SCHIZOPHRENIA

1 Schizophrenia cannot be understood without understanding despair.
R. D. Laing (1927–) British psychiatrist.
The Divided Self

2 Schizophrenic behaviour is a special strategy that a person invents in order to live in an unlivable situation.
R. D. Laing
The Divided Self

3 If you talk to God, you are praying; if God talks to you, you have schizophre-

nia. If the dead talk to you, you are a spiritualist; if God talks to you, you are a schizophrenic.
Thomas Szasz (1920–   ) US psychiatrist.
The Second Sin

SCIENCE

1   On 13 September 1765 people in fields near Luce, in France, saw a stone-mass drop from the sky after a violent thunderclap. The great physicist Lavoisier, who knew better than any peasant that this was impossible, reported to the Academy of Science that the witnesses were mistaken or lying. The Academy would not accept the reality of meteorites until 1803.
Fortean Times

2   Science has nothing to be ashamed of, even in the ruins of Nagasaki.
Jacob Brownowski (1908–74) British scientist and mathematician.
Science and Human Values

3   Putting on the spectacles of science in expectation of finding the answer to everything looked at signifies inner blindness.
J. Frank Dobie (1888–1964)
The Voice of Coyote, Introduction

4   The content of physics is the concern of physicists, its effect the concern of all men.
Friedrich Dürrenmatt (1921–   ) Swiss writer.
The Physicists

5   Facts are not science – as the dictionary is not literature.
Martin H. Fischer (1879–1962)
Fischerisms (Howard Fabing and Ray Marr)

6   Thus I saw that most men only care for science so far as they get a living by it, and that they worship even error when it affords them a subsistence.
Johann Wolfgang von Goethe (1749–1832) German poet, dramatist, and scientist.
Conversations with Goethe (Johann Peter Eckermann)

7   Science is not to be regarded merely as a storehouse of facts to be used for material purposes, but as one of the great human endeavours to be ranked with arts and religion as the guide and expression of man's fearless quest for truth.
Sir Richard Arman Gregory (1864–1952)
The Harvest of a Quiet Eye (Alan L. Mackay)

8   The World would be a safer place,
    If someone had a plan,
    Before exploring Outer Space,

To find the Inner Man.
E. Y. Harburg (1896–1981) US songwriter.

9   Science is the father of knowledge, but opinion breeds ignorance.
    Hippocrates (c. 460 BC–c. 377 BC) Greek physician.
    The Canon Law, IV

10 Science . . . commits suicide when it adopts a creed.
    Thomas Huxley (1825–95) British biologist.
    Darwiniana, 'The Darwin Memorial'

11 Reason, Observation, and Experience – the Holy Trinity of Science.
    Robert G. Ingersoll (1833–99) US lawyer and agnostic.
    The Gods

12 Many persons nowadays seem to think that any conclusion must be very sci-
    entific if the arguments in favor of it are derived from twitching of frogs' legs
    – especially if the frogs are decapitated – and that – on the other hand –
    any doctrine chiefly vouched for by the feelings of human beings – with
    heads on their shoulders – must be benighted and supersititious.
    William James (1842–1910) US psychologist and philosopher.
    Pragmatism

13 Let both sides seek to invoke the wonders of science instead of its terrors.
    Together let us explore the stars, conquer the deserts, eradicate disease, tap
    the ocean depths, and encourage the arts and commerce.
    John F. Kennedy (1917–63) US statesman.
    Inaugural Address, 20 Jan 1961

14 We have genuflected before the god of science only to find that it has given
    us the atomic bomb, producing fears and anxieties that science can never
    mitigate.
    Martin Luther King (1929–68) US Black Civil rights leader.
    Strength through Love, Ch. 13

15 Science conducts us, step by step, through the whole range of creation, until
    we arrive, at length, at God.
    Marguerite of Valois (1553–1615)
    Memoirs (1594–1600), Letter XII

16 We have no right to assume that any physical laws exist, or if they have ex-
    isted up to now, that they will continue to exist in a similar manner in the
    future.
    Max Planck (1858–1947) German physicist.
    The Universe in the Light of Modern Physics

17 Science may be described as the art of systematic over-simplification.
    Karl Popper (1902–   ) Austrian-born British philosopher.
    Remark, Aug 1982

18 Science without conscience is the death of the soul.
    François Rabelais (c. 1494–1553) French writer.

19 The simplest schoolboy is now familiar with truths for which Archimedes
    would have sacrificed his life.
    Ernest Renan (1823–92) French philosopher and theologian.
    Souvenirs d'enfance et de jeunesse

20 Science is what you know, philosophy is what you don't know.
    Bertrand Russell (1872–1970) British philosopher.

21 When we have found how the nucleus of atoms are built-up we shall have
    found the greatest secret of all – except life. We shall have found the basis
    of everything – of the earth we walk on, of the air we breathe, of the sun-
    shine, of our physical body itself, of everything in the world, however great
    or however small – except life.
    Ernest Rutherford (1871–1937) British physicist.
    Passing Show 24

22 People must understand that science is inherently neither a potential for good
    nor for evil. It is a potential to be harnessed by man to do his bidding.
    Glenn T. Seaborg (1912–) US physicist.
    Associated Press interview with Alton Blakeslee, 29 Sept 1964

23 Science is always wrong. It never solves a problem without creating ten more.
    George Bernard Shaw (1856–1950) Irish dramatist and critic.

24 The technology of medicine has outrun its sociology.
    Henry E. Sigerist (1891–1957)
    Medicine and Human Welfare, Ch. 3

25 Science is the great antidote to the poison of enthusiasm and superstition.
    Adam Smith (1723–90) Scottish economist.
    The Wealth of Nations, Bk. V, Ch. 1

26 Science robs men of wisdom and usually converts them into phantom beings
    loaded up with facts.
    Miguel de Unamuno y Jugo (1864–1936) Spanish writer and philosopher.
    Essays and Soliloquies

27 Whenever science makes a discovery, the devil grabs it while the angels are
    debating the best way to use it.
    Alan Valentine

SENILITY

1 Body and mind, like man and wife, do not always agree to die together.
    Charles C. Colton (c. 1780–1832) British churchman and writer.
    Lacon, Vol. I, Ch. 324

2   Bodily decay is gloomy in prospect, but of all human contemplations the most
    abhorrent is body without mind.
    Thomas Jefferson (1743–1826) US statesman.
    Letter to John Adams, 1 Aug 1816

3   That ends this strange eventful history,
    Is second childishness and mere oblivion,
    Sans teeth, sans eye, sans taste, sans everything.
    William Shakespeare (1564–1616) English dramatist and poet.
    As You Like It, II:7

SEX

1   Writing about erotics is a perfectly respectable function of medicine, and
    about the way to make the woman enjoy sex; these are an important part of
    reproductive physiology.
    Avicenna (Ibn Sina; 980–1037)
    Sex in Society (Alex Comfort)

2   Physically, a man is a man for a much longer time than a woman is a
    woman.
    Honoré de Balzac (1799–1850) French writer.
    The Physiology of Marriage

3   Sexuality is the lyricism of the masses.
    Charles Baudelaire (1821–67) French poet.
    Journaux intimes, 93

4   He said it was artificial respiration but now I find I'm to have his child.
    Anthony Burgess (John Burgess Wilson; 1917–   ) British writer.
    Inside Mr. Enderby

5   I'll wager you that in 10 years it will be fashionable again to be a virgin.
    Barbara Cartland (1902–   ) British romantic novelist.
    The Observer, 'Sayings of the Week', 20 June 1976

6   I said 10 years ago that in 10 years time it would be smart to be a virgin.
    Now everyone is back to virgins again.
    Barbara Cartland
    The Observer, 'Sayings of the Week', 12 July 1987

7   The pleasure is momentary, the position ridiculous and the expense
    damnable.
    Earl of Chesterfield (1694–1773) English statesman.
    Nature, 1970, 227, 772

8   No more about sex, it's too boring. Everyone's got one. Nastiness is a real
     stimulant though—but poor honest sex, like dying, should be a private matter.
     Laurence Durrell (1912–) British novelist and poet.
     Prospero's Cell, Ch. 1

9   You think intercourse is a private act; it's not, it's a social act. Men are sexu-
     ally predatory in life; and women are sexually manipulative. When two indi-
     viduals come together and leave their gender outside the bedroom door, then
     they make love. If they take it inside with them, they do something else, be-
     cause society is in the room with them.
     Andrea Dworkin US feminist.
     Intercourse

10   For all the pseudo-sophistication of twentieth-century sex theory, it is still as-
     sumed that a man should make love as if his principal intention was to peo-
     ple the wilderness.
     Germaine Greer (1939–) Australian-born British writer and feminist.

11   No sex is better than bad sex.
     Germaine Greer
     Attrib.

12   People will insist . . . on treating the *mons Veneris* as though it were Mount
     Everest.
     Aldous Huxley (1894–1964) British writer.
     Eyeless in Gaza, Ch. 30

13   There's nothing wrong with going to bed with somebody of your own sex.
     People should be very free with sex—they should draw the line at goats.
     Elton John (1947–) British rock pianist and singer.

14   The discussion of the sexual problem is, of course, only the somewhat crude
     beginning of a far deeper question, namely, that of the psychic of human re-
     lationship between the sexes. Before this later question the sexual problem
     pales into significance.
     C. G. Jung (1875–1961) Swiss psychologist.
     Bartlett's Unfamiliar Quotations (Leonard Louis Levinson)

15   To be solemn about the organs of generation is only possible to someone
     who, like Lawrence, has deified the will and denied the spirit.
     Hugh Kingsmill
     Referring to D. H. Lawrence
     Tread Softly for You Tread on My Jokes (Malcolm Muggeridge)

16   Who would not be curious to see the lineaments of a man who, having him-
     self been twice married wished that mankind were propagated like trees.
     Charles Lamb (1775–1834) British essayist.
     New Monthly Magazine, Jan 1826
     Referring to Sir Thomas Browne

17   You mustn't think I advocate perpetual sex. Far from it. Nothing nauseates
     me more than promiscuous sex in and out of season.
     D. H. Lawrence (1885–1930) British writer.
     Letter to Lady Ottoline Morrell, 22 Dec 1928
     Referring to *Lady Chatterley's Lover*

18   Making love is the sovereign remedy for anguish.
     Frédérick Leboyer (1918–) French obstetrician.
     Birth without Violence

19   No sex without responsibility.
     Lord Longford (1905–) British politician and social reformer.
     Observer, 3 May 1954

20   The reproduction of mankind is a great marvel and mystery. Had God con-
     sulted me in the matter, I should have advised him to continue the genera-
     tion of the species by fashioning them of clay.
     Martin Luther (1483–1546) German Protestant reformer.

21   Men have broad and large chests, and small narrow hips, and more under-
     standing than women, who have but small and narrow breasts, and broad
     hips, to the end they should remain at home, sit still, keep house, and bear
     and bring up children.
     Martin Luther
     Table-Talk, 'Of Marriage and Celibacy'

22   Effusion of semen represents the strength of the body and its life . . . when-
     ever it is emitted to excess, the body becomes consumed, its strength termi-
     nates and its life perishes. . . . He who immerses himself in sexual intercourse
     will be assailed by premature ageing, his strength will wane, his eyes will
     weaken, and a bad odour will emit from his mouth and his armpits, his teeth
     will fall out and many other maladies will afflict him.
     Maimonides (Moses ben Maimon; 1135–1204) Spanish-born Jewish philosopher
     and physician.
     Mishreh Torah

23   If sex is such a natural phenomenon, how come there are so many books on
     how to?
     Bette Midler US actress and comedienne.

24   Sex is one of the nine reasons for reincarnation . . . The other eight are
     unimportant.
     Henry Miller (1891–1980) US novelist.
     Big Sur and the Oranges of Hieronymus Bosch

25   When she saw the sign 'Members Only' she thought of him.
     Spike Milligan (1918–) British comic actor and writer.
     Puckoon

26 The orgasm has replaced the Cross as the focus of longing and the image of fulfilment.
Malcolm Muggeridge (1903–) British writer and editor.
The Most of Malcolm Muggeridge, 'Down with Sex'

27 I know it does make people happy but to me it is just like having a cup of tea.
Cynthia Payne (1934–) British housewife.
After her acquittal on a charge of controlling prostitutes in a famous 'sex-for-luncheon-vouchers' case, 8 Nov 1987

28 Love is two minutes fifty-two seconds of squishing noises. It shows your mind isn't clicking right.
Johnny Rotten (1957–) British punk musician.
Daily Mirror, 1983

29 Love as a relation between men and women was ruined by the desire to make sure of the legitimacy of the children.
Bertrand Russell (1872–1970) British philosopher.
Marriage and Morals

30 His excessive emphasis on sex was due to the fact that in sex alone he was compelled to admit that he was not the only human being in the universe. It was so painful that he conceived of sex relations as a perpetual fight in which each is attempting to destroy the other.
Bertrand Russell
Autobiography
Referring to D.H. Lawrence

31 Civilized people cannot fully satisfy their sexual instinct without love.
Bertrand Russell
Marriage and Morals, 'The Place of Love in Human Life'

32 Is it not strange that desire should so many years outlive performance?
William Shakespeare (1564–1616) English dramatist and poet.
Henry IV, Part Two, II:4

33 Is Sex Necessary?
James Thurber and E. B. White (1894–1961 and 1899–) US writers, humorists, and cartoonists.
Title of a book

34 Once: a philosopher; twice: a pervert!
Voltaire (François-Marie Arouet; 1694–1778) French writer and philosopher.
Turning down an invitation to an orgy, having attended one the previous night for the first time
Attrib.

35 All this fuss about sleeping together. For physical pleasure I'd sooner go to the dentist any day.
Evelyn Waugh (1903–66) British writer.

36 The mind can also be an erogenous zone.
Raquel Welch (1940–) US film star.
Colombo's Hollywood (J.R. Colombo)

37 Freud found sex an outcast in the outhouse and left it in the living room an honored guest.
W. Beran Wolfe
The Great Quotations (George Seldes)
Referring to Sigmund Freud

SIGHT

1 Our sight is the most perfect and most delightful of all our senses. It fills the mind with the largest variety of ideas, converses with its objects at the greatest distance, and continues the longest in action without being tired or satiated with its proper enjoyments.
Joseph Addison (1672–1719) British essayist.
The Spectator, 411

SKIN

1 Dermatology is the best speciality. The patient never dies – and never gets well.
Anonymous

2 Skin is like wax paper that holds everything in without dripping.
Art Linkletter (1912–) Canadian-born US radio and television personality.
A Child's Garden of Misinformation, 5

3 Woollen clothing keeps the skin healthy.
Venetian proverb

SLEEP

1 The amount of sleep required by the average person is just five minutes more.
Anonymous

2 Oh sleep! it is a gentle thing,
Beloved from pole to pole!
Samuel Taylor Coleridge (1772–1834) British poet.
The Rime of the Ancient Mariner, V

3   Sleep is that golden chaine that ties health and our bodies together.
    Thomas Dekker (c. 1572–c. 1632) English dramatist.
    The Guls Horn-Booke, Ch. 2

4   Health is the first muse, and sleep is the condition to produce it.
    Ralph Waldo Emerson (1803–82) US poet and essayist.
    Uncollected Lectures, 'Resources'

5   Sleep is when all the unsorted stuff comes flying out as from a dustbin upset
    in a high wind.
    William Golding (1911–) British novelist.
    Pincher Martin

6   Sleep is gross, a form of abandonment, and it is impossible for anyone to
    awake and observe its sordid consequences save with a faint sense of recent
    dissipation, of minute personal disquiet and remorse.
    Patrick Hamilton
    Slaves of Solitude

7   Sleep and watchfulness, both of them, when immoderate, constitute disease.
    Hippocrates (c. 460 BC–c. 377 BC) Greek physician.
    Aphorisms, II

8   The beginning of health is sleep.
    Irish proverb

9   I have, all my life long, been lying till noon; yet I tell all young men, and
    tell them with great sincerity, that nobody who does not rise early will ever
    do any good.
    Samuel Johnson (1709–84) British lexicographer and writer.
    Tour to the Hebrides (J. Boswell)

10 The average, healthy, well-adjusted adult gets up at seven-thirty in the morn-
    ing feeling just plain terrible.
    Jean Kerr (1923–) US dramatist, screenwriter, and humorist.
    Please Don't Eat the Daisies, 'Where Did You Put the Aspirin?'

11 Those no-sooner-have-I-touched-the-pillow people are past my comprehension.
    There is something bovine about them.
    J. B. Priestley (1894–1984) British novelist.
    All About Ourselves

12 Early to bed and early to rise, makes a man healthy, wealthy and wise.
    Proverb

13 One hour's sleep before midnight, is worth two after.
    Proverb

14 Sleep is better than medicine.
    Proverb

15 Our foster nurse of nature is repose.
William Shakespeare (1564–1616) English dramatist and poet.
King Lear, IV

16 Sleep that knits up the ravell'd sleeve of care,
The death of each day's life, sore labour's bath,
Balm of hurt minds, great nature's second course,
Chief nourisher in life's feast.
William Shakespeare
Macbeth, II:2

17 Sleep's the only medicine that gives ease.
Sophocles (c. 496 BC–406 BC) Greek dramatist.
Philoctetes, 766

18 Of all the soft, delicious functions of nature this is the chiefest; what a happiness it is to man, when the anxieties and passions of the day are over.
Laurence Sterne (1713–68) Irish-born English novelist.

19 Early to rise and early to bed makes a male healthy and wealthy and dead.
James Thurber (1894–1961) US writer, cartoonist, and humorist.
Fables for Our Time, 'The Shrike and the Chipmunks'

20 That sweet, deep sleep, so close to tranquil death.
Virgil (Publius Vergilius Maro; 70 BC–19 BC) Roman poet.
Aeneid, VI

21 I haven't been to sleep for over a year. That's why I go to bed early. One needs more rest if one doesn't sleep.
Evelyn Waugh (1903–66) British novelist.
Decline and Fall, Pt. II, Ch. 3

SLIMMING

1 My advice if you insist on slimming: Eat as much as you like – just don't swallow it.
Harry Secombe (1921–) Welsh singer, actor, and comedian.
Daily Herald, 5 Oct 1962

SMOKING

1 Caution: Cigarette Smoking May Be Hazardous to Your Health.
Anonymous
Statement required on cigarette packets

2   The Elizabethan age might be better named the beginning of the smoking era.
    J. M. Barrie (1860–1937) British novelist and dramatist.
    My Lady Nicotine

3   Certainly not – if you don't object if I'm sick.
    Thomas Beecham (1879–1961) British conductor.
    Attrib.
    When asked whether he minded if someone smoked in a non-smoking compartment

4   Tobacco, divine, rare, superexcellent tobacco, which goes far beyond all their panaceas, potable gold, and philosopher's stones, a sovereign remedy to all diseases.
    Robert Burton (1577–1640) English scholar and explorer.
    Anatomy of Melancholy

5   Smokers, male and female, inject and excuse idleness in their lives every time they light a cigarette.
    Colette (Sidonie Gabrielle Claudine Colette; 1873–1954) French novelist.
    Earthly Paradise, 'Freedom'

6   I have seen many a man turn his gold into smoke, but you are the first who has turned smoke into gold.
    Elizabeth I (1533–1603) Queen of England.
    Speaking to Sir Walter Raleigh

7   What smells so? Has somebody been burning a Rag, or is there a Dead Mule in the Back yard? No, the Man is Smoking a Five-Cent Cigar.
    Eugene Field (1850–95) US poet and journalist.
    The Tribune Primer, 'The Five-Cent Cigar'

8   Tobacco surely was designed
    To poison, and destroy mankind.
    Philip Freneau (1752–1832) US poet.
    Poems, 'Tobacco'

9   What a blessing this smoking is! perhaps the greatest that we owe to the discovery of America.
    Arthur Helps (1813–75) British historian.
    Friends in Council

10 Tobacco is a dirty weed. I like it.
    It satisfies no normal need. I like it.
    It makes you thin, it makes you lean,
    It takes the hair right off your bean.
    It's the worst darn stuff I've ever seen.
    I like it.
    Graham Lee Hemminger (1896–1949)
    Penn State Froth, Nov 1915

11   But when I don't smoke I scarcely feel as if I'm living. I don't feel as if I'm
     living unless I'm killing myself.
     Russell Hoban
     Turtle Diary, Ch. 7

12   A custom loathsome to the eye, hateful to the nose, harmful to the brain,
     dangerous to the lungs, and in the black, stinking fume thereof, nearest re-
     sembling the horrible Stygian smoke of the pit that is bottomless.
     James I (1566–1625) King of England.
     A Counterblast to Tobacco

13   Smoking . . . is a shocking thing, blowing smoke out of our mouths into other
     people's mouths, eyes and noses, and having the same thing done to us.
     Samuel Johnson (1709–84) English lexicographer and writer.
     Tour to the Hebrides (James Boswell)

14   Neither do thou lust after that tawney weed tobacco.
     Ben Jonson (1573–1637) English dramatist.
     Bartholomew Fair, II:6

15   Ods me, I marvel what pleasure or felicity they have in taking their roguish
     tobacco. It is good for nothing but to choke a man, and fill him full of
     smoke and embers.
     Ben Jonson
     Every Man in His Humour, III:5

16   The tobacco business is a conspiracy against womanhood and manhood. It
     owes its origin to that scoundrel Sir Walter Ralegh, who was likewise the
     founder of American slavery.
     Dr. John Harvey Kellogg
     Tobacco

17   A woman is only a woman, but a good cigar is a smoke.
     Rudyard Kipling (1865–1936) Indian-born British writer and poet.
     The Betrothed

18   It is now proved beyond doubt that smoking is one of the leading causes of
     statistics.
     Fletcher Knebel
     Reader's Digest, Dec 1961

19   This very night I am going to leave off tobacco! Surely there must be some
     other world in which this unconquerable purpose shall be realized. The soul
     hath not her generous aspirings implanted in her in vain.
     Charles Lamb (1775–1834) British essayist.
     Letter to Thomas Manning, 26 Dec 1815

20   No matter what Aristotle and all philosophy may say, there's nothing like to-

bacco. 'Tis the passion of decent folk; he who lives without tobacco isn't worthy of living.
Molière (Jean-Baptiste Poquelin; 1622–73) French dramatist.
Don Juan, ou le festin de Pierre, I:1

21   My doctor has always told me to smoke. He even explains himself: 'Smoke, my friend. Otherwise someone else will smoke in your place.'
Erik Satie (1866–1925) French composer.
Mémoires d'un amnésique

22   I have every sympathy with the American who was so horrified by what he had read of the effects of smoking that he gave up reading.
Henry G. Strauss
Quotations for Speakers and Writers (A. Andrews)

23   I asked a coughing friend of mine why he doesn't stop smoking. 'In this town it wouldn't do any good,' he explained. 'I happen to be a chain breather.'
Robert Sylvester (1907–75) US writer.
Attrib.

24   We shall not refuse tobacco the credit of being sometimes medical, when used temperately, though an acknowledged poison.
Jesse Torrey (1787–1834)
The Moral Instructor, Pt. IV

25   When I was young, I kissed my first woman, and smoked my first cigarette on the same day. Believe me, never since have I wasted any more time on tobacco.
Arturo Toscanini (1867–1957) Italian conductor.

26   To cease smoking is the easiest thing I ever did. I ought to know because I've done it a thousand times.
Mark Twain (Samuel L. Clemens; 1835–1910) US writer.

27   There are people who strictly deprive themselves of each and every eatable, drinkable and smokable which has in any way acquired a shady reputation. They pay this price for health. And health is all they get for it.
Mark Twain

28   Tobacco drieth the brain, dimmeth the sight, vitiateth the smell, hurteth the stomach, destroyeth the concoction, disturbeth the humors and spirits, corrupteth the breath, induceth a trembling of the limbs, exsiccateth the windpipe, lungs, and liver, annoyeth the milt, scorcheth the heart, and causeth the blood to be adjusted.
Tobias Venner (1577–1660)
Via Recta ad Vitam Longam

29 A cigarette is the perfect type of a perfect pleasure. It is exquisite, and it
    leaves one unsatisfied. What more can one want?
    Oscar Wilde (1854–1900) Irish-born British dramatist.
    The Picture of Dorian Gray, Ch. 6

SNORING

1 Laugh and the world laughs with you; snore and you sleep alone.
   Anthony Burgess (John Burgess Wilson; 1917–) British writer.
   Inside Mr. Enderby

2 There ain't no way to find out why a snorer can't hear himself snore.
   Mark Twain (Samuel L. Clemens; 1835–1910) US writer.
   Tom Sawyer Abroad, Ch. 10

STATISTICS

1 Medical statistics are like a bikini. What they reveal is interesting but what
   they conceal is vital.
   Anonymous

2 There are two kinds of statistics, the kind you look up and the kind you
   make up.
   Rex Stout (1886–1975) US writer.
   Death of a Doxy, Ch. 9

STRESS

1 Despair is better treated with hope, not dope.
   Richard Asher (1912–)
   Lancet, I:954, 1958

2 Every little yielding to anxiety is a step away from the natural heart of man.
   Japanese proverb

3 Worry affects circulation, the heart and the glands, the whole nervous sytem,
   and profoundly affects the heart. I have never known a man who died from
   overwork, but many who died from doubt.
   Charles H. Mayo (1865–1939) US physician.
   Bartlett's Unfamiliar Quotations (Leonard Louis Levinson)

SUFFERING

1 Rather suffer than die is man's motto.
   Jean de La Fontaine (1621–95) French poet.
   Fables, I, 'La Mort et le Bûcheron'

2 A man who fears suffering is already suffering from what he fears.
Michel de Montaigne (1533–92) French essayist and moralist.
Essays, III

SUICIDE

1 To run away from trouble is a form of cowardice and, while it is true that
the suicide braves death, he does it not for some noble object but to escape
some ill.
Aristotle (384 BC–322 BC) Greek philosopher and scientist.
Nicomachean Ethics, 3

2 If I had the use of my body I would throw it out of the window.
Samuel Beckett (1906–) Irish novelist and dramatist.
Malone Dies

3 If you must commit suicide . . . always contrive to do it as decorously as possi-
ble; the decencies, whether of life or of death, should never be lost sight of.
George Borrow (1803–81)
Lavengro, Ch. 23

4 As soon as one does not kill oneself, one must keep silent about life.
Albert Camus (1913–60) French existentialist writer.
Notebooks 1935–1942, 1

5 There is but one truly serious philosophical problem and that is suicide. Judging whether life is or is not worth living amounts to answering the fundamental question of philosophy.
Albert Camus
The Myth of Sisyphus

6 To attempt suicide is a criminal offense. Any man who, of his own will, tries
to escape the treadmill to which the rest of us feel chained incites our envy,
and therefore our fury. We do not suffer him to go unpunished.
Alexander Chase (1926–) US journalist.
Perspectives

7 The strangest whim has seized me. . . . After all
I think I will not hang myself today.
G. K. Chesterton (1874–1936) British writer.
A Ballade of Suicide

8 Suicide is the worst form of murder, because it leaves no opportunity for
repentance.
John Churton Collins (1848–1908)
Life and Memoirs of John Churton Collins, Appendix VII (L. C. Collins)

9 There are many who dare not kill themselves for fear of what the neighbours might say.
Cyril Connolly (1903–74) British writer and critic.
The Unquiet Grave

10 Self-destruction is the effect of cowardice in the highest extreme.
Daniel Defoe (c. 1659–1731) English journalist and writer.
An Essay Upon Projects, 'Of Projectors'

11 My work is done. Why wait?
George Eastman (1854–1932) US inventor and industrialist.
His suicide note

12 The prevalence of suicide is a test of height in civilization; it means that the population is winding up its nervous and intellectual system to the utmost point of tension and that sometimes it snaps.
Havelock Ellis (1859–1939) British psychologist.

13 Suicide is not a remedy.
James A. Garfield (1831–81) US statesman.
Inaugural address, 4 Mar 1881

14 However great a man's fear of life . . . suicide remains the courageous act, the clear-headed act of a mathematician. The suicide has judged by the laws of chance – so many odds against one, that to live will be more miserable than to die. His sense of mathematics is greater than his sense of survival.
Graham Greene (1904–   ) British novelist.
The Comedians, I

15 Hatred and the feeling of solidarity pay a high psychological dividend. The statistics of suicide show that, for noncombatants at least, life is more interesting in war than in peace.
W. R. Inge (1860–1954) British writer and churchman.
The End of an Age, Ch. 3

16 I take it that no man is educated who has never dallied with the thought of suicide.
William James (1842–1910) US psychologist and philosopher.

17 I have been half in love with easeful Death.
John Keats (1795–1821) British poet.
Ode to a Nightingale

18 Suicide is something on its own. It seems to me to be a flight by which man hopes to recover Paradise Lost instead of trying to deserve Heaven.
Paul-Louis Landsberg (1901–43)
The Experience of Death and the Moral Problem of Suicide

19 Nature puts upon no man an unbearable burden; if her limits be exceeded,

man responds by suicide. I have always respected suicide as a regulator of
nature.
Emil Ludwig (1881–1948)
I Believe (Clifton Fadiman)

20   The thought of suicide is a great source of comfort: with it a calm passage is
to be made across many a bad night.
Friedrich Wilhelm Nietzsche (1844–1900) German philosopher.
Jenseits von Gut und Böse

21   When you go to drown yourself always take off your clothes, they may fit
your wife's next husband.
Gregory Nunn

22   Razors pain you
Rivers are damp;
Acids stain you;
And drugs cause cramp.
Guns aren't lawful;
Nooses give;
Gas smells awful;
You might as well live.
Dorothy Parker (1893–1967) US humorous writer.
Enough Rope, 'Resumé'

23   No one ever lacks a good reason for suicide.
Cesare Pavese (1908–1950) Italian writer.

24   Amid the sufferings of life on earth, suicide is God's best gift to man.
Pliny the Elder (23 AD–79 AD) Roman scholar.
Natural History, 2

25   When you're between any sort of devil and the deep blue sea, the deep blue
sea sometimes looks very inviting.
Terence Rattigan (1911–77) British dramatist.
The Deep Blue Sea

26   How many people have wanted to kill themselves, and have been content
with tearing up their photograph!
Jules Renard (1864–1910) French writer.
Journal

27   It is against the law to commit suicide in this man's town . . . although what
the law can do to a guy who commits suicide I am never able to figure out.
Damon Runyon (1884–1946) US writer.
Guys and Dolls

28   Dost thou not see my baby at my breast

That sucks the nurse asleep?
William Shakespeare (1564–1616) English dramatist and poet.
Antony and Cleopatra, V:2
Holding the asp to her breast

29 A still small voice spake unto me,
    'Thou art so full of misery,
    Were it not better not to be?'
    Alfred, Lord Tennyson (1809–92) British poet.
    The Two Voices

30 Not that suicide always comes from madness. There are said to be occasions
    when a wise man takes that course: but, generally speaking, it is not in an
    access of reasonableness that people kill themselves.
    Voltaire (François Marie Arouet; 1694–1778) French writer and philosopher.
    Letter to James Marriott, 1767

31 There is no refuge from confession but suicide; and suicide is confession.
    Daniel Webster (1782–1852) US statesman.
    *The Murder of Captain Joseph White: Argument on the Trial of John Francis
    Knapp*

SURGEONS

1 The egotistical surgeon is like a monkey; the higher he climbs the more you
   see of his less attractive features.
   Anonymous

2 The operation was successful – but the patient died.
   Anonymous

3 Tree surgeons are taught to wear safety belts so they won't fall out of
   patients.
   Anonymous

4 The glory of surgeons is like that of actors, who exist only in their lifetime
   and whose talent is no longer appreciable once they have disappeared.
   Honoré de Balzac (1799–1850) French novelist.
   The Atheist's Mass

5 I never say of an operation that it is without danger.
   August Bier (1861–1949)

6 The feasibility of an operation is not the *best* indication for its performance.
   Henry, Lord Cohen of Birkenhead (1900–)
   Annals of the Royal College of Surgeons of England 6:3, 1950

7   Surgery does the ideal thing – it separates the patient from his disease. It
puts the patient back to bed and the disease in a bottle.
Logan Clendening (1884–1945)
Modern Methods of Treatment, Ch. 1

8   But after all, when all is said and done, the king of all topics is operations.
Irvin S. Cobb (1876–1944) US humorist and journalist.
Speaking of Operations

9   My lectures were highly esteemed, but I am of the opinion my operations
rather kept down my practice.
Sir Astley Paston Cooper (1768–1841)
Bulletin of the New York Academy of Medicine, 5:155, 1929 (F. H. Garrison)

10   I have made many mistakes myself; in learning the anatomy of the eye I dare
say, I have spoiled a hatful; the best surgeon, like the best general, is he who
makes the fewest mistakes.
Sir Astley Paston Cooper
Lectures on Surgery

11   A good surgeon operates with his hand, not with his heart.
Alexandre Dumas père (1802–70) French novelist and dramatist.

12   Or, take a surgical operation.
In consultation with the doctor and the surgeon,
In going to bed in the nursing home,
In talking to the matron you are still the subject,
The centre of reality. But, stretched on the table,
You are a piece of furniture in a repair shop
For those who surround you, the masked actors;
All there is of you is your body
All the 'you' is withdrawn.
T. S. Eliot (1888–1965) US-born British poet and dramatist.
The Cocktail Party, I:1

13   The practice of medicine is a thinker's art the practice of surgery a plumber's.
Martin H. Fischer (1879–1962)
Aphorism

14   Surgery is the ready motion of steady and experienced hands.
Galen (fl. 2nd century) Greek physician and scholar.
Definitiones Medicae, XXXV

15   Before undergoing a surgical operation arrange your temporal affairs – you
may live.
Remy de Gourmont (1858–1915)

16 The only weapon with which the unconscious patient can immediately retaliate upon the incompetent surgeon is haemorrhage.
William Stewart Halsted (1852–1922)
Bulletin of the Johns Hopkins Hospital, 23:191, 1912

17 The lancet was the magician's wand of the dark ages of medicine.
Oliver Wendell Holmes (1809–94) US writer and physician.
Medical Essays, 'Some of My Early Teachers'

18 The first attribute of a surgeon is an insatiable curiosity.
Russell John Howard (1875–1942)
The Hip, Ch. 2 (F. G. St. Clair Strange)

19 The most important person in the operating theatre is the patient.
Russell John Howard
The Hip, Ch. 3 (F. G. St. Clair Strange)

20 Speed in operating should be the achievement, not the aim, of every surgeon.
Russell John Howard
The Hip, Ch. 9 (F. G. St. Clair Strange)

21 In surgery eyes first and most fingers next and little; tongue last and least.
Sir George Murray Humphry (1820–96)

22 Speaking of the importance of draining abscesses he referred to the time when he was called to Balmoral to operate upon Queen Victoria for an axillary abscess and playfully said, 'Gentlemen, I am the only man who has ever stuck a knife in the Queen.'
J. R. Leeson
Lister as I Knew Him
Referring to Joseph Lister

23 A possible apprehension now is that the surgeon be sometimes tempted to supplant instead of aiding Nature.
Henry Maudsley (1835–1918)

24 A vain surgeon is like a milking stool, of no use except when sat upon.
Robert Tuttle Morris (1857–1945)

25 The greatest triumph of surgery today . . . lies in finding ways for avoiding surgery.
Robert Tuttle Morris
Doctors versus Folks, Ch. 3

26 Any fool can cut off a leg – it takes a surgeon to save one.
George G. Ross (1834–92)

27 Lose a leg rather than life.
Proverb

28 The best surgeon is he that has been well hacked himself.
Proverb

29 Can honour set to a leg? No. Or an arm? No. Or take away the grief of a wound? No. Honour hath no skill in surgery, then? No.
William Shakespeare (1564–1616) English dramatist and poet.
Henry IV, Part One, V:1

30 In surgery all operations are recorded as successful if the patient can be got out of the hospital or nursing home alive, though the subsequent history of the case may be such as would make an honest surgeon vow never to recommend or perform the operation again.
George Bernard Shaw (1856–1950) Irish dramatist and critic.
The Doctor's Dilemma, 'Preface on Doctors'

31 Now it cannot be too often repeated that when an operation is once performed, nobody can ever prove that it was unnecessary. If I refuse to allow my leg to be amputated, its mortification and my death may prove that I was wrong; but if I let the leg go, nobody can ever prove that it would not have mortified had I been obstinate. Operation is therefore the safe side for the surgeon as well as the lucrative side.
George Bernard Shaw
The Doctor's Dilemma, 'Preface on Doctors'

32 When *I* take up assassination, I shall start with the surgeons in this city and work *up* to the gutter.
Dylan Thomas (1914–53) Welsh poet.
The Doctor and the Devils, 88

33 Human beings, yes, but not surgeons.
Rudolph Virchow (1821–1902) German pathologist.
Anekdotenschatz (H. Hoffmeister)
Answering a query as to whether human beings could survive appendectomy, which had recently become a widespread practice

34 The operation wasn't bad. I quite enjoyed the trip up from my room to the operating parlors, as a closely confined person does enjoy any sort of outing. The morphine had loosened my tongue, and while we waited in the corridor for the surgeon to arrive, the orderly and I let down our hair and had a good chat about fishing tackle.
E. B. White (1899–   ) US journalist and humorous writer.
The Second Tree from the Corner, 'A Weekend with the Angels'

35 In a good surgeon, a hawk's eye: a lion's heart: and a lady's hand.
Leonard Wright
Display of Dutie

T

TEACHING

1   If I were summing up the qualities of a good teacher of medicine, I would enumerate human sympathy, moral and intellectual integrity, enthusiasm, and ability to talk, in addition, of course, to knowledge of his subject.
Anonymous

2   A professor is a gentleman who has a different opinion.
August Bier (1861–1949)
Aphorism

3   If there weren't so many professors, medicine would be much easier.
August Bier
Aphorism

4   A teacher is paid to teach, not to sacrifice rats and hamsters.
Edward A. Gall (1906–)
Journal of Medical Education, 36:275, 1961

5   A good clinical teacher is himself a Medical School.
Oliver Wendell Holmes (1809–94) US writer and physician.
Medical Essays, 'Scholastic and Bedside Teaching'

6   The bedside is always the true center of medical teaching.
Oliver Wendell Holmes
Medical Essays, 'Scholastic and Bedside Teaching'

7   Those of us who have the duty of training the rising generation of doctors . . . must not inseminate the virgin minds of the young with the tares of our own fads. It is for this reason that it is easily possible for teaching to be too 'up to date'. It is always well, before handing the cup of knowledge to the young, to wait until the froth has settled.
Sir Robert Hutchison (1871–1960)
British Medical Journal, 1:995, 1925

8   The safest thing for a patient is to be in the hands of a man engaged in teaching medicine. In order to be a teacher of medicine the doctor must always be a student.
Charles H. Mayo (1865–1939) US physician.
Proceedings of the Staff Meetings of the Mayo Clinic, 2:233, 1927

9   I have learned since to be a better student, and to be ready to say to my fellow students 'I do not know.'
    Sir William Osler (1849–1919) Canadian physician.
    Aequanimitas, with Other Addresses, 'After Twenty-Five Years'

10 I desire no other epitaph – no hurry about it, I may say – than the statement that I taught medical students in the wards, as I regard this as by far the most useful and important work I have been called upon to do.
    Sir William Osler
    Aequanimitas, with Other Addresses, 'The Fixed Period'

11 The successful teacher is no longer on a height, pumping knowledge at high pressure into passive receptacles. . . . He is a senior student anxious to help his juniors.
    Sir William Osler
    The Student Life

12 If they are not interested in the care of the patient, in the phenomena of disease in the sick, they should not be in the clinical department of medicine, since they cannot teach students clinical medicine.
    Maurice B. Strauss (1904–74)
    Medicine, 43:619, 1964

TEETH

1   Removing the teeth will cure something, including the foolish belief that removing the teeth will cure everything.
    Anonymous

2   DENTIST, n. A prestidigitator who, putting metal into your mouth, pulls coins out of your pocket.
    Ambrose Bierce (1842–c. 1914) US writer and journalist.
    The Devil's Dictionary

3   Every Tooth in a Man's Head is more valuable than a Diamond.
    Miguel de Cervantes (1547–1616) Spanish novelist.
    Don Quixote, Pt. I, Ch. 4

4   It is necessary to clean the teeth frequently, more especially after meals, but not on any account with a pin, or the point of a penknife, and it must never be done at table.
    St. Jean Baptiste de la Salle (1651–1719)
    The Rules of Christian Manners and Civility, I

5   I find that most men would rather have their bellies opened for five hundred dollars than have a tooth pulled for five.
    Martin H. Fischer (1879–1962)
    Fischerisms (Howard Fabing and Ray Marr)

6   For years I have let dentists ride roughshod over my teeth: I have been
    sawed, hacked, chopped, whittled, bewitched, bewildered, tattooed, and
    signed on again; but this is cuspid's last stand.
    S. J. Perelman (1904–79) US humorous writer.
    Crazy Like a Fox, 'Nothing but the Tooth'

7   I'll dispose of my teeth as I see fit, and after they've gone, I'll get along. I
    started off living on gruel, and by God, I can always go back to it again.
    S. J. Perelman
    Crazy Like a Fox, 'Nothing but the Tooth'

8   Certain people are born with natural false teeth.
    Robert Robinson (1927–) British writer and broadcaster.
    BBC radio programme, *Stop the Week*, 1977

9   He that sleeps feels no the toothache.
    William Shakespeare (1564–1616) English dramatist and poet.
    Cymbeline

10 For there was never yet philosopher
    That could endure the toothache patiently.
    William Shakespeare
    Much Ado About Nothing, V:1

11 The man with toothache thinks everyone happy whose teeth are sound.
    George Bernard Shaw (1856–1950) Irish dramatist and critic.
    Man and Superman, 'Maxims for Revolutionists'

12 Sweet things are bad for the teeth.
    Jonathan Swift (1667–1746) Anglo-Irish priest, poet, and satirist.
    Polite Conversation, Dialogue II

13 Adam and Eve had many advantages, but the principal one was that they es-
    caped teething.
    Mark Twain (Samuel L. Clemens; 1835–1910) US writer.
    The Tragedy of Pudd'nhead Wilson, Ch. 4

14 To lose a lover or even a husband or two during the course of one's life can
    be vexing. But to lose one's teeth is a catastrophe.
    Hugh Wheeler (1912–) British-born US writer.
    A Little Night Music

THEORY

1   Medical theories are most of the time even more peculiar than the facts
    themselves.
    August Bier (1861–1949)
    Aphorism

2   Don't confuse *hypothesis* and *theory*. The former is a possible explanation; the

latter, the correct one. The establishment of theory is the very purpose of science.
Martin H. Fischer (1879–1962)
Fischerisms (Howard Fabing and Ray Marr)

3   Those who are enamoured of practice without science are like a pilot who goes into a ship without rudder or compass and never has any certainty where he is going.
Practice should always be based upon a sound knowledge of theory.
Leonardo da Vinci (1452–1519) Italian artist, sculptor, architect, and engineer.
The Notebooks of Leonardo da Vinci (Edward MacCurdy)

4   Physicians are inclined to engage in hasty generalizations. Possessing a natural or acquired distinction, endowed with a quick intelligence, an elegant and facile conversation . . . the more eminent they are . . . the less leisure they have for investigative work . . . . Eager for knowledge . . . they are apt to accept too readily attractive but inadequately proven theories.
Louis Pasteur (1822–95) French scientist.
Etudes sur la bière, Ch. 3

5   In making theories always keep a window open so that you can throw one out if necessary.
Béla Schick (1877–1967) Austrian pediatrician.
Aphorisms and Facetiae of Béla Schick (I.J. Wolf)

THINKING

1   It would not be at all a bad thing if the elite of the medical world would be a little less clever, and would adopt a more primitive method of thinking, and reason more as children do.
George Groddeck (1866–1934)
The Book of the It, Letter XII

2   One of the worst diseases to which the human creature is liable is its disease of thinking.
John Ruskin (1819–1900) British art critic and social reformer.
The Political Economy of Art, 'A Joy For Ever'

3   Thinking is the most unhealthy thing in the world, and people die of it just as they die of any other disease.
Oscar Wilde (1854–1900) Irish-born British writer and wit.
The Decay of Lying

TIME

1   Time is the great physician.
Benjamin Disraeli, Lord Beaconsfield (1804–81) British statesman.
Henrietta Temple, Bk. VI, Ch. 9

2   A physician can sometimes parry the scythe of death, but has no power over
    the sand in the hourglass.
    Hester Lynch Piozzi (Mrs. Henry Thrale; 1741–1821) British writer.
    Letter to Fanny Burney, 22 Nov 1781

3   Time cures the sick man, not the ointment.
    Proverb

4   The physician's best remedy is *Tincture of Time!*
    Béla Schick (1877–1967) Austrian pediatrician.
    Aphorisms and Facetiae of Béla Schick (I.J. Wolf)

5   Time heals what reason cannot.
    Seneca (c. 4 BC–65 AD) Roman writer.
    Agamemnon

6   Time carries all things, even our wits, away.
    Virgil (Publius Vergilius Maro; 70 BC–19 BC) Roman poet.
    Eclogues, IX

TRANSPLANTS

1   The human body is the only machine for which there are no spare parts.
    Hermann M. Biggs (1859–1923)
    Radio talk

TREATMENT

1   I haven't asked you to make me young again. All I want is to go on getting
    older.
    Konrad Adenauer (1876–1967) German statesman.
    Attrib.
    Replying to his doctor

2   Difficult as it may be to cure, it is always easy to poison and to kill.
    Elisha Bartlett (1804–55)
    Philosophy of Medical Science, Pt. II, Ch. 16

3   Every hospital should have a plaque in the physicians' and students' en-
    trances: 'There are some patients whom we cannot help, there are none
    whom we cannot harm.'
    Arthur L. Bloomfield (1888–1962)
    Personal communication after iatrogenic tragedy, c. 1930–36

4   Some day when you have time, look into the business of prayer, amulets,

baths and poultices, and discover for yourself how much valuable therapy the profession has cast on the dump.
Martin H. Fischer (1879–1962)
Fisherisms (Howard Fabing and Ray Marr)

5 Never forget that it is not a pneumonia, but a pneumonic man who is your patient. Not a typhoid fever, but a typhoid man.
Sir William Withey Gull (1816–90)
Published Writings, Memoir II

6 Medicines are nothing in themselves, if not properly used, but the very hands of the gods, if employed with reason and prudence.
Herophilus (fl. 300 BC) Greek physician.

7 As to diseases, make a habit of two things – to help, or at least to do no harm.
Hippocrates (c. 460 BC–c. 377 BC) Greek physician.
Epidemics, Bk. I

8 *Nature*, in medical language, as opposed to Art, means trust in the reactions of the living system against ordinary normal impressions.
Art, in the same language, as opposed to Nature, means an intentional resort to extraordinary abnormal impressions for the relief of disease.
Oliver Wendell Holmes (1809–94) US writer and physician.
Medical Essays, 'Currents and Counter-Currents in Medical Science'

9 Diagnosis precedes treatment.
Russell John Howard (1875–1942)
The Hip (F. G. St. Clair Strange)

10 The treatment with poison medicines comes from the West.
Huang Ti (The Yellow Emperor; 2697 BC–2597 BC)
Nei Ching Su Wên, Bk. 4

11 After thirty years' practice, I am fully convinced that two-thirds of all my patients would have recovered without the use of physic, or the attendance of a physician.
Christoph Wilhelm Hufeland (1762–1836)

12 Treat the man who is sick and not a Greek name.
Abraham Jacobi (1830–1919)
Bulletin of the New York Academy of Medicine, 4:1003, 1928

13 In the old-fashioned days when a man got sick he went to the family doctor and said he was sick. The doctor gave him a bottle of medicine. He took it home and drank it and got well.
On the bottle was written, 'Three times a day in water.' The man drank it three times a day the first day, twice the second day, and once the third day. On the fourth day he forgot it. But that didn't matter. He was well by that time . . . .

Such medicine was, of course, hopelessly unscientific, hopelessly limited.
Death could beat it round every corner. But it was human, gracious, kindly.
Stephen Leacock (1869–1944) English-born Canadian economist and humorist.
The Leacock Roundabout, 'The Doctor and the Contraption'

14 You know that medicines when well used restore health to the sick: they will
be well used when the doctor together with his understanding of their nature
shall understand also what man is, what life is, and what constitution and
health are. Know these well and you will know their opposites; and when
this is the case you will know well how to devise a remedy.
Leonardo da Vinci (1452–1519) Italian artist, sculptor, architect, and engineer.
Codice Atlantico, 270

15 When people's ill, they comes to I,
I physics, bleeds, and sweats 'em;
Sometimes they live, sometimes they die.
What's that to I? I lets 'em.
John Coakley Lettsom (1744–1815)
On Dr. Lettsom, by Himself

16 Keep up the spirits of your patient with the music of the viol and the psal-
tery, or by forging letters telling of the death of his enemies or (if he be a
cleric) by informing him that he has been made a bishop.
Henri de Mondeville
Bartlett's Unfamiliar Quotations (Leonard Louis Levinson)

17 It is the patient rather than the case which requires treatment.
Robert Tuttle Morris (1857–1945)
Doctors versus Folks, Ch. 2

18 Medicine is not yet liberated from the medieval idea that disease is the result
of sin and must be expiated by mortification of the flesh.
Sir George W. Pickering (1904–)
Resident Physician, II (No. 9): 71, 1965

19 In treating a patient, let your first thought be to strengthen his natural
vitality.
Rhazes (Ar-Razi; 850–923) Persian physician and philosopher.

20 The physician cannot prescribe by letter the proper time for teating or bath-
ing; he must feel the pulse.
Seneca (c. 4 BC–65 AD) Roman writer.
Epistulae ad Lucilium, XII

TRUTH

1   Before you tell the 'truth' to the patient, be sure you know the 'truth,' and
    that the patient wants to hear it.
    Richard Clarke Cabot (1868–1939)
    Journal of Chronic Diseases, 16:443, 1963

2   What I tell you three times is true.
    Lewis Carroll (Charles Lutwidge Dodgson; 1832–98) British writer.
    The Hunting of the Snark

3   The great glory of modern medicine is that it regards nothing as essential but
    the truth.
    Burton J. Hendrick (1870–1949)

4   Truths without exception are not the truths most commonly met with in
    medicine.
    Peter Mere Latham (1789–1875) US poet and essayist.
    Diseases of the Heart, Lecture III

5   How is it that in medicine Truth is thus measured out to us in fragments,
    and we are never put in trust of it *as a whole*?
    Peter Mere Latham
    General Remarks on the Practice of Medicine, Ch. 13

TUBERCULOSIS

1   There is a dread disease which so prepares its victim, as it were, for death;
    . . . a disease in which death and life are so strangely blended, that death
    takes a glow and hue of life, and life the gaunt and grisly form of death – a
    disease which medicine never cured, wealth warded off, or poverty could
    boast exemption from – which sometimes moves in giant strides, and some-
    times at a tardy sluggish pace, but, slow or quick, is ever sure and certain.
    Charles Dickens (1812–70) British novelist.
    Nicholas Nickleby, Ch. 49

2   Decay and disease are often beautiful, like the pearly tear of the shellfish and
    the hectic glow of consumption.
    Henry David Thoreau (1817–62) US writer.
    Journal, 11 June 1852

3   I would like to remind those responsible for the treatment of tuberculosis that
    Keats wrote his best poems while dying of this disease. In my opinion he
    would never have done so under the influence of modern chemotherapy.
    Arthur M. Walker (1896–1955)
    Walkerisms (Julius L. Wilson)

U

ULCERS

1   The view that a peptic ulcer may be the hole in a man's stomach through
    which he crawls to escape from his wife has fairly wide acceptance.
    J. A. D. Anderson (1926–   )
    A New Look at Social Medicine

2   I don't have ulcers; I give them.
    Harry Cohn (1891–1958) US film producer.

3   Unfortunately, only a small number of patients with peptic ulcer are finan-
    cially able to make a pet of an ulcer.
    William James Mayo (1861–1934) US surgeon.
    Journal of the American Medical Association, 79:19, 1922

UNIVERSE

1   There is no reason to assume that the universe has the slightest interest in
    intelligence – or even in life. Both may be random accidental by-products of
    its operations like the beautiful patterns on a butterfly's wings. The insect
    would fly just as well without them.
    Arthur C. Clarke (1917–   ) British science-fiction writer.
    The Lost Worlds of 2001

2   My suspicion is that the universe is not only queerer than we suppose, but
    queerer than we *can* suppose.
    J. B. S. Haldane (1892–1964) British geneticist.
    Possible Worlds, 'On Being the Right Size'

V

VACCINATION

1 Vaccination is the medical sacrament corresponding to baptism.
Samuel Butler (1835–1902) British writer.

2 If he is to be allowed to let his children go unvaccinated, he might as well be allowed to leave strychnine lozenges about in the way of mine.
T. H. Huxley (1825–95) British biologist.
Method and Results, 'Administrative Nihilism'
Referring to his next-door neighbour

3 The scepticism that appeared, even among the most enlightened of medical men when my sentiments on the important subject of the cow-pox were first promulgated, was highly laudable. To have admitted the truth of a doctrine, at once so novel and so unlike anything that ever had appeared in the annals of medicine, without the test of the most rigid scrutiny, would have bordered upon temerity.
Edward Jenner (1749–1823) English physician.
A Continuation of Facts and Observations Relative to the Variolae Vaccinae, or Cow-Pox

VASECTOMY

1 Vasectomy means not ever having to say you're sorry.
Larry Adler (1914–) US harmonica player and entertainer.
Before his vasectomy operation

VENEREAL DISEASE

1 Despite a lifetime of service to the cause of sexual liberation I have never caught a venereal disease, which makes me feel rather like an arctic explorer who has never had frostbite.
Germaine Greer (1939–) Australian-born British writer and feminist.
The Observer, 'Sayings of the Week', 4 Mar 1973

2 Two minutes with Venus, two years with mercury.
J. Earle Moore (1892–1957)
Aphorism

VIRGINITY

1   Virginity is rather a state of mind.
     Maxwell Anderson (1888–1959)
     Elizabeth the Queen, II:3

VITALISM

1   I also suspect that many workers in this field and related fields have been
     strongly motivated by the desire, rarely actually expressed, to refute vitalism.
     Francis H. C. Crick (1916–) British biophysicist.
     Referring to molecular biology
     British Medical Bulletin, 21:183, 1965

2   As long as vitalism and spiritualism are open questions so long will the gate-
     way of science be open to mysticism.
     Rudolf Virchow (1821–1902) German pathologist.
     Bulletin of the New York Academy of Medicine, 4:994, 1928

VIVISECTION

1   I would rather that any white rabbit on earth should have the Asiatic cholera
     twice than that I should have it just once.
     Irvin S. Cobb (1876–1944)

2   Vivisection . . . is justifiable for real investigations on physiology; but not for
     mere damnable and detestable curiosity.
     Charles Darwin (1809–22) British life scientist.
     Letter, 22 Mar 1871

3   There are a few honest antivivisectionists. . . . I have not met any of them,
     but I am quite prepared to believe that they exist.
     J. B. S. Haldane (1892–1964) British geneticist.
     Possible Worlds, 'Some Enemies of Science'

4   I know not, that by living dissections any discovery has been made by which
     a single malady is more easily cured.
     Samuel Johnson (1709–84) English lexicographer and writer.
     The Idler, No. 17, 5 Aug 1758

5   There are people who do not object to eating a mutton chop–people who do
     not even object to shooting a pheasant with the considerable chance that it
     may be only wounded and may have to die after lingering in pain, unable to
     obtain its proper nutriment–and yet who consider it something monstrous to

introduce under the skin of a guinea pig a little inoculation of some microbe
to ascertain its action. These seem to me to be most inconsistent views.
Joseph, Lord Lister (1827–1912) British surgeon.
British Medical Journal, 1:317, 1897

6   Like following life through creatures you dissect,
    You lose it in the moment you detect.
    Alexander Pope (1688–1744) English poet.
    Moral Essays, I

W-X-Y

WOMEN

1   A maiden at college, named Breeze,
    Weighed down by B.A.s and M.D.s
    Collapsed from the strain.
    Said her doctor, 'It's plain
    You are killing yourself by degrees!'
    Anonymous

2   It is almost a pity that a woman has a womb.
    Anonymous
    Woman and Nature (Susan Griffin)

3   Science seldom renders men amiable; women, never.
    Edmone-Pierre Chanvot de Beauchêne (1748–1824)
    Maximes, réflexions et pensées diverses

4   One is not born a woman, one becomes one.
    Simone de Beauvoir (1908–86) French writer.
    The Second Sex, Ch. 2

5   It is in great part the anxiety of being a woman that devastates the feminine
    body.
    Simone de Beauvoir
    Womansize (Kim Chernin)

6   It is obvious that we cannot instruct women as we do men in the science of
    medicine; we cannot carry them into the dissecting room.
    Walter Channing
    *Remarks on the Employment of Females as Practitioners in Midwifery, by a Physi-
    cian*

7   Mother love, particularly in America, is a highly respected and much publi-
    cized emotion and when exacerbated by gin and bourbon it can become ex-
    tremely formidable.
    Noël Coward (1899–1973) British dramatist.
    Future Indefinite

8   What is woman? – only one of Nature's agreeable blunders.
    Hannah Cowley (1743–1809) English poet and dramatist.
    Who's the Dupe?, II

9   Women are most fascinating between the ages of thirty-five and forty, after

they have won a few races and know how to pace themselves. Since few women ever pass forty, maximum fascination can continue indefinitely.
Christian Dior (1905–57) French fashion designer.
Colliers Magazine, 10 June 1955

10   A woman should be an illusion.
Ian Fleming (1908–64) British journalist and writer.
Life of Ian Fleming (John Pearson)

11   What does a woman want?
Sigmund Freud (1856–1939) Austrian psychoanalyst.

12   The only bodily organ which is really regarded as inferior is the atrophied penis, a girl's clitoris.
Sigmund Freud
'The Dissection of the Psychical Personality'

13   Women are equal because they are not different any more.
Erich Fromm (1910–80) US psychologist and philosopher.
The Art of Loving

14   The female breast has been called 'the badge of femininity'. In order for the breast to be aesthetically pleasing, it should be a relatively firm, full breast which stands out from the chest wall and states with certainty, 'I am feminine'.
John Ransom Lewis, Jnr. M.D.
Atlas of Aesthetic Plastic Surgery

15   Other books have been written by men physicians. . . . One would suppose in reading them that women possess but one class of physical organs, and that these are always diseased. Such teaching is pestiferous, and tends to cause and perpetuate the very evils it professes to remedy.
Mary Ashton Livermore (c. 1820–1905) US writer.
What Shall We Do with Our Daughters?, Ch. 2

16   The Professor of Gynaecology . . . began his course of lectures as follows: Gentlemen, woman is an animal that micturates once a day, defecates once a week, menstruates once a month, parturates once a year and copulates whenever she has the opportunity.
W. Somerset Maugham (1874–1965) British writer and doctor.
A Writer's Notebook

17   The moral world of the sick-bed explains in a measure some of the things that are strange in daily life, and the man who does not know sick women does not know women.
S. Weir Mitchell (1829–1914)
Doctor and Patient, Introduction

18   When a woman becomes a scholar there is usually something wrong with her
      sexual organs.
      Friedrich Nietzche (1844–1900) German philosopher.
      Bartlett's Unfamiliar Quotations (Leonard Louis Levinson)

19   When I think of women, it is their hair which first comes to my mind. The
      very idea of womanhood is a storm of hair . . . .
      Friedrich Nietzsche
      My Sister and I

20   God created woman. And boredom did indeed cease from that moment – but
      many other things ceased as well! Woman was God's *second* mistake.
      Friedrich Nietzsche
      The Antichrist

21   The surgical cycle in woman: Appendix removed, right kidney hooked up,
      gall-bladder taken out, gastro-enterostomy, clean sweep of uterus and adnexa.
      Sir William Osler (1849–1919) Canadian physician.
      Sir William Osler: Aphorisms (William B. Bean)

22   Six men give a doctor less to do than one woman.
      Proverb

23   The doctors said at the time that she couldn't live more than a fortnight,
      and she's been trying ever since to see if she could. Women are so
      opinionated.
      Saki (Hector Hugh Munro; 1870–1916) British writer.
      Reginald on Women

24   Women exist in the main solely for the propagation of the species.
      Arthur Schopenhauer (1788–1860) German philosopher.

25   A determining point in the history of gynecology is to be found in the fact
      that sex plays a more important part in the life of woman than in that of
      man, and that she is more burdened by her sex.
      Henry E. Sigerist (1891–1957)
      American Journal of Obstetrics and Gynecology 42:714, 1941

26   An ailing woman lives forever.
      Spanish proverb

27   Womanhood is the great fact in her life; wifehood and motherhood are but
      incidental relations.
      Elizabeth Stanton (1815–1902) US suffragette.
      History of Woman Suffrage (with Susan B. Anthony and Mathilda Gage), Vol.
      I

28   Woman is unrivaled as a wet nurse.
      Mark Twain (Samuel L. Clemens; 1835–1910) US writer.

WORK

1 Work is the grand cure of all the maladies and miseries that ever beset
  mankind.
  Thomas Carlyle (1795–1881) Scottish historian and essayist.
  Inaugural address at Edinburgh University, 1866

2 Employment is nature's physician, and is essential to human happiness.
  Galen (fl. 2nd century) Greek physician and scholar.

3 . . . she had always found occupation to be one of the best medicines for an
  afflicted mind . . . .
  Eliza Leslie (1787–1858)
  Pencil Sketches; or, Outlines of Character and Manners, 'Constance Allerton; or
  the Mourning Suits'

4 Temperance and labour are the two real physicians of man: labour sharpens
  his appetite and temperance prevents his abusing it.
  Jean Jacques Rousseau (1712–78) French philosopher.
  Emile, Bk. I

WORRY

1 Before the cherry orchard was sold everybody was worried and upset, but as
  soon as it was all settled finally and once for all, everybody calmed down,
  and felt quite cheerful.
  Anton Chekhov (1860–1904) Russian dramatist.
  The Cherry Orchard, IV

2 When I look back on all these worries I remember the story of the old man
  who said on his deathbed that he had had a lot of trouble in his life, most of
  which had never happened.
  Winston Churchill (1874–1965) British statesman.
  Their Finest Hour

3 Worrying is the most natural and spontaneous of all human functions. It is
  time to acknowledge this, perhaps even to learn to do it better.
  Lewis Thomas (1913–) US pathologist.
  More Notes of a Biology Watcher, 'The Medusa and the Snail'

WOUNDS

1 What deep wounds ever closed without a scar?
  George Gordon, Lord Byron (1788–1824) British poet.

2   Bind up their wounds—but look the other way.
    W. S. Gilbert (1836–1911) British dramatist.
    Princess Ida, III

3   A wound heals but the scar remains.
    Proverb

X-RAYS

1   X-RAYS: Their moral is this—that a right way of looking at things will see
    through almost anything.
    Samuel Butler (1835–1902) British writer.
    Note-Books, Vol. V

2   A device which enables us to see how the bones in the back room are doing.
    Don Quinn
    Bartlett's Unfamiliar Quotations (Leonard Louis Levinson)

YOUTH

1   A stage between infancy and adultery.
    Anonymous

2   No young man believes he shall ever die.
    William Hazlitt (1778–1830) British essayist.
    The Monthly Magazine, Mar 1827

3   Is is the malady of our age that the young are so busy teaching us that they
    have no time left to learn.
    Eric Hoffer (1902–) US writer.

4   A majority of young people seem to develop mental arteriosclerosis forty years
    before they get the physical kind.
    Aldous Huxley (1894–1964) British writer.
    Writers at Work: Second Series
    Interview

5   Youth is in itself so amiable, that were the soul as perfect as the body, we
    could not forbear adoring it.
    Marie de Sévigné (1626–96) French letter-writer.
    Letter to her daughter

6   Youth is a malady of which one becomes cured a little every day.
    Benito Mussolini (1883–1945) Italian dictator.
    Said on his 50th birthday

7   In the spring . . . your lovely Chloë lightly turns to one mass of spots.
    Ronald Searle (1920–) British cartoonist.
    The Terror of St Trinian's, Ch. 7

8   I would there were no age between ten and three-and-twenty, or that youth
    would sleep out the rest; for there is nothing in the between but getting
    wenches with child, wronging the ancientry, stealing, fighting.
    William Shakespeare (1564–1616) English dramatist and poet.
    The Winter's Tale, III

9   Youth is a wonderful thing. What a crime to waste it on children.
    George Bernard Shaw (1856–1950) Irish dramatist and critic.

10 No wise man ever wished to be younger.
    Jonathan Swift (1667–1745) Anglo-Irish priest, satirist, and poet.
    Thoughts on Various Subjects, Moral and Diverting

KEYWORD INDEX

Man . . . is halfway between an a. and a god
MANKIND, 16
the a. from which he is descended EVOLUTION, 26
The exception is a naked a. MANKIND, 21
aphrodisiac The moon is nothing But a circumambulating a. FERTILITY, 1
apoplexy A. is an affection of the head JARGON, 21
apothecary A. n. The physician's accomplice DRUGS, 4
apothicaries A good Kitchen is a good A. shop
HEALTHY EATING, 2
appearances you must preserve a. SANITY, 1
appendicitis chronic remunerative a. MEDICAL FEES, 13
appetite Doth not the a. alter? OLD AGE, 39
Illness isn't the only thing that spoils the a. HEALTHY
EATING, 26
apple An a. a day HEALTHY LIVING, 24
An a. a day keeps the doctor away. PREVENTIVE
MEDICINE, 3
Archimedes The . . . schoolboy is now familiar with
truths for which A. SCIENCE, 19
architect from the point of view of the hygienist, the
physician, the a. HOSPITALS, 3
the a. can only advise MISTAKES, 8
art exercises his a. with caution DOCTORS, 103
Let him learn their a. properly MISTAKES, 6
Medicine is a natural a. HISTORY OF MEDICINE, 3
Science and a. are only too often a superior kind of
dope NARCOTICS, 12
This aspect of . . . medicine has been designated as
the a. DOCTORS AND PATIENTS, 7
arteries A man is as old as his a. AGE, 14
arteriosclerosis young people seem to develop mental
a. YOUTH, 4
ascertainable the a. laws of the science of life are approximative MEDICINE, 5
aspirations The young have a. MEMORY, 2
aspirin from the humble a. DRUGS, 19
if tranquillizers could be bought as easily and
cheaply as a. they would be consumed DRUGS, 13
aspirings The soul hath not her generous a.
SMOKING, 19
assembly an ingenious a. of portable plumbing
MANKIND, 20
asthma A. is a disease that has practically the same
symptoms as passion ASTHMA, 1
asylum An a. for the sane would be empty in
America. SANITY, 5
Had there been a Lunatic A. in the suburbs of Jerusalem MENTAL ILLNESS, 16
I have myself spent nine years in a lunatic a.
PSYCHIATRY, 4
The place where optimism most flourishes is the lunatic a. MENTAL ILLNESS, 17
asylums the a. can hold the sane people SANITY, 7
ate I a. faster. HEALTHY EATING, 13
authorities Patients consult so-called a.
CONSULTANTS, 4
authority a top hat to give him A. DOCTORS, 4
it can maintain a wise infidelity against the a. of his
instructors MEDICAL STUDENTS, 9

babies If men had to have b. BIRTH, 8
putting milk into b. CHILD CARE, 6
baby Every b. born into the world BABIES, 2
Hanging head downwards between cliffs of bone, was
the b. PREGNANCY, 1
my b. at my breast SUICIDE, 28
bacillus Oh, powerful b. GERMS, 4

back any of you at the b. who do not hear me
DISABILITY, 1
bacteriologists staff of b. CONSULTANTS, 2
balanced Food is an important part of a b. diet
HEALTHY EATING, 12
bald The most delightful advantage of being b.
BALDNESS, 1
baldness There is more felicity on the far side of b.
BALDNESS, 4
There's one thing about b. BALDNESS, 3
barren There is nothing encourageth a woman sooner
to be b. BIRTH, 17
bastard It serves me right for putting all my eggs in
one b. ABORTION, 3
bath B. . . . once a week to avoid being a public
menace HYGIENE, 2
bathe B. early every day and sickness will avoid you.
HYGIENE, 4
bats His father's sister had b. in the belfry and was
put away. MENTAL ILLNESS, 37
beast Every man has a wild b. within him.
MANKIND, 11
beastliness called in our schools 'b.' MASTURBATION, 2
beautifully Living well and b. and justly HEALTHY
LIVING, 28
beauty Health is b. HEALTH, 19
bed A man of sixty has spent twenty years in b.
LIFE, 1
bedside not in the lecture room, but at the b.
MEDICAL STUDENTS, 7
beefsteak a b. prevents it. PREVENTIVE MEDICINE, 8
behaviourism Of course, B. 'works'. PSYCHIATRY, 6
being look on him again as a whole b. PATIENTS, 6
To kill a human b. EUTHANASIA, 5
beings We tolerate shapes in human b. BODY, 7
belfry His father's sister had bats in the b. and was
put away. MENTAL ILLNESS, 37
bell never send to know for whom the b. tolls
DEATH, 24
best b. of life is but intoxication DRINKING, 11
betake And so I b. myself to that course BLINDNESS, 7
better I am getting b. and b. PSYCHOLOGY, 3;
REMEDIES, 9
bilious to be b. with. LIVER, 1
biology The separation of psychology from the premises of b. PSYCHOLOGY, 7
birds except that the b. might eat them DRUGS, 8
birth an environment equally fit for b., growth,
work, healing, and dying HEALTHY LIVING, 14
B., and copulation, and death LIFE AND DEATH, 5
B. may be a matter of a moment BIRTH, 15
From b. to age eighteen, a girl needs good parents
AGE, 16
Man's main task in life is to give b. to himself
BIRTH, 13
Our b. is but a sleep and a forgetting BIRTH, 22
The history of man for the nine months preceding
his b. PREGNANCY, 2
The memory of b. LIFE AND DEATH, 6
There is no cure for b. and death LIFE, 21
To hinder a b. is merely speedier man-killing
ABORTION, 5
bite 'You should not b. the hand that feeds you.'
HEALTHY EATING, 25
bladder master of his soul, Is servant to his b.? OLD
AGE, 5
blank Pain – has an Element of B. PAIN, 6
blessing a b. that money cannot buy. HEALTH, 22

health! the b. of the rich! the riches of the poor
HEALTH, 10

blessings The trained nurse has become one of the
great b. of humanity   NURSING, 7

blind b. as those who won't see   BLINDNESS, 8
b. in their own cause   BLINDNESS, 9
I have a right to be b. sometimes   BLINDNESS, 6
In the Country of the B.   BLINDNESS, 10
It is not miserable to be b.   BLINDNESS, 3

blindness it is miserable to be incapable of enduring
b.   BLINDNESS, 3
My b. is my sight   BLINDNESS, 2

blood How does the heart pump b.   BODY, 5
it touches a man that his b. is sea water
ENVIRONMENT, 4
leeches have red b.   BLOOD, 1
men with our own real body and b.   BODY, 6

bloodiness The sink is the great symbol of the b. of
family life   FAMILY, 3; NEUROSIS, 10

blunders The b. of a doctor   MISTAKES, 2

bodies I will abstain from . . . abusing the b. of man
or woman,   MEDICAL ETHICS, 5
Minds like b., will often fall into a pimpled, ill-conditioned state   MIND, 2
Our minds are lazier than our b.   MIND AND BODY, 7
Sleep is that golden chaine that ties health and our
b. together   SLEEP, 3
what happens in our b. is directed toward a useful
end.   MEDICINE, 10
You may house their b. but not their souls   CHILD
CARE, 9

body A b. seriously out of equilibrium   MENTAL
ILLNESS, 42
A healthy b. is the guest-chamber of the soul
BODY, 1
All there is of you is your b.   SURGEONS, 12
A man ought to handle his b. like the sail of a ship
HEALTHY LIVING, 23
an intimate knowledge of the human b.   MEDICINE, 26
a sound mind in a sound b.   HEALTH, 11; HEALTHY
LIVING, 17
B. and mind, . . . , do not always agree to die to-
gether   SENILITY, 1
B. and soul cannot be separated for purposes of
treatment   HOLISTIC MEDICINE, 8
by whom it is impossible to make ourselves understood: our b.   BODY, 12
cure the infirmities of the b.   DIAGNOSIS, 6
Disease is not of the b.   DISEASE, 15
diseases as isolated disturbances in a healthy b.
DISEASE, 1
fear made manifest on the b.   CHRISTIAN SCIENCE, 2
Happiness is beneficial for the b.   MIND, 14
Her b. dissected by fiendish men   DISSECTION, 1
her long struggle between mind and b.   ANOREXIA, 2
If I had the use of my b.   SUICIDE, 2
If the b. be feeble, the mind will not be strong
HOLISTIC MEDICINE, 5
It is fear made manifest on the b.   MIND AND BODY, 1
it leaves them nothing but b.   DISEASE, 9
knows the properties of the human b.   DOCTORS, 103
medicine . . . the knowledge of the loves and desires
of the b.   MEDICINE, 44
men with our own real b. and blood   BODY, 6
mind and b. must develop in harmonious propor-
tions   EXERCISE, 7
Our b. is a machine for living   REMEDIES, 19
Pain of mind is worse than pain of b.   MENTAL
ILLNESS, 49

So long as the b. is affected through the mind
HOMEOPATHY, 6
The b. is not a permanent dwelling   BODY, 13
The b. is truly the garment of the soul   BODY, 3
The b. must be repaired   HOLISTIC MEDICINE, 11
The human b. is a machine   BODY, 9
The human b. is like a bakery HOLISTIC MEDICINE, 12
The human b. is private property.   RESEARCH, 29
the human b. is sacred   BODY, 14
The human b. is the best picture of the human soul
BODY, 15
The human b. is the only machine   TRANSPLANTS, 1
the human psyche lives in indissoluble union with
the b.   PSYCHOLOGY, 7
The mind grows sicker than the b.   MENTAL ILLNESS, 35
The mind has great influence over the b.   MIND AND
BODY, 6
the most abhorrent is b. without mind   SENILITY, 2
the mysteries of the human b.   MEDICINE, 22
the observations of the b. in health and disease
NATURE, 8
the physicians separate the soul from the b. HOLISTIC
MEDICINE, 9
There is more wisdom in your b.   BODY, 11
the secrets of the structure of the human b.
DEATH, 27
We have rudiments of reverence for the human b.
MIND AND BODY, 3
Well in b. But sick in mind   HOLISTIC MEDICINE, 10
when the soul is oppressed so is the b.   HOLISTIC
MEDICINE, 7

body-snatcher B., . . . One who supplies the young
physicians   DISSECTION, 3

bomb god of science . . . has given us the atomic b.
SCIENCE, 14

bones how the b. in the back room are doing
X-RAYS, 2

Borgia makes good use of the B. effect   DRUGS, 3

born A man is not completely b.   BIRTH, 11
As soon as man is b.   DEATH, 54
for joy that a man is b. into the world   BIRTH, 4
he is not conscious of being b.   LIFE AND DEATH, 10
It is as natural to die as to be b.   BIRTH, 2
one of woman b.   BIRTH, 18
We are all b. mad   MENTAL ILLNESS, 3

botanize Physician art thou? . . . One that would peep
and b.   DOCTORS, 111

bowels a good reliable sett ov b. iz wurth more tu a
man   CONSTIPATION, 1
separating disorders of the chest from disorders of
the b.   BODY, 2
spin conversation thus incessantly out of thy own b.
HYPOCHONDRIA, 9

brain B., n. An apparatus with which we think that
we think   BRAIN, 2
It is good to rub and polish our b.   BRAIN, 9
My b.: it's my second favourite organ   BRAIN, 1
our b. is a mystery   BRAIN, 4
Pure symmetry of the b.   BRAIN, 7
that most perfect and complex of computers the
human b.   MEDICAL STUDENTS, 12
the biggest b. of all the primates   MEN, 2
The b. has muscles for thinking   BRAIN, 8
The b. is a wonderful organ   BRAIN, 6
The b. is not an organ to be relied upon   BRAIN, 3
The b. is the organ of longevity   BRAIN, 10
the human b. is a device   BRAIN, 5
the universe, the reflection of the structure of the b.
BRAIN, 4

Tobacco drieth the b. SMOKING, 28
brains many b. and many hands are needed
RESEARCH, 36
those who practise with their b. DOCTORS, 61
brass Make it compulsory for a doctor using a b.
plate DOCTORS, 89
brat than it is to turn one b. into a decent human
being CHILD CARE, 12
bread One swears by wholemeal b. HEALTHY EATING, 10
breakdown One of the symptoms of approaching nervous b. MENTAL ILLNESS, 39
breast my baby at my b. SUICIDE, 28
The female b. has been called 'the badge of femininity' WOMEN, 14
breasts women, who have but small and narrow b.
SEX, 21
breath The first b. is the beginning of death
DEATH, 56
breather I happen to be a chain b. SMOKING, 23
breathing Keep b. LONGEVITY, 10
breeding God-like in our . . . b. of . . . plants and animals EVOLUTION, 75
brewery The b. is the best drugstore DRINKING, 33
brightness To pass away ere life hath lost its b.
DEATH, 30
British B. loathe the middle-aged MIDDLE AGE, 11
but we are B. – thank God HOMOSEXUALITY, 3
brook b. no contradiction DOCTORS, 107
buildings to design features in such b. that are posi-
tively healing HOSPITALS, 4
burden that one is a b. to the host BODY, 13
burst She b. while drinking a seidlitz powder;
DEATH, 6
business limit to what one can learn about normal b.
transactions POST-MORTEM, 1

calories the only thing that matters is c. HEALTHY
EATING, 10
cancer C.'s a Funny Thing: CANCER, 1
there are several chronic diseases more destructive to
life than c., none is more feared CANCER, 2
to give up everything that scientists have linked to
c. HYPOCHONDRIA, 1
cant Popular psychology is a mass of c. PSYCHOLOGY, 4
carcinoma To sing of rectal c. CANCER, 3
cardio-sclerotic We have here an antique c.
JARGON, 12
care Effective health c. depends on self-c. HEALTH
CARE, 1
For want of timely c. MISTAKES, 1
People who are always taking c. of their health are
like misers, HYPOCHONDRIA, 15
Sleep that knits up the ravell'd sleave of c. SLEEP, 16
The first C. in building of Cities ENVIRONMENT, 1
case It is not a c. we are treating PATIENTS, 1
the patient not only as a c. but also as an individual
DOCTORS, 16
cases a narrative of the special c. of his patients CASE
HISTORY, 2
castle A neurotic is the man who builds a c. in the
air. PSYCHIATRY, 46
cataclysm Out of their c. but one poor Noah Dare
hope to survive CONCEPTION, 2
catastrophe to lose one's teeth is a c. TEETH, 14
Catholic quite lawful for a C. woman to avoid pregnancy by . . . mathematics CONTRACEPTION, 6
cause A reckoning up of the c. often solves the malady CURES, 11

has to know the c. of the ailment before he can
cure it DIAGNOSIS, 18
to attribute to a single c. that which is the product
of several DIAGNOSIS, 14
cavity filling his last c. DENTISTS, 1
celery two thousand people crunching c. at the same
time HEALTHY EATING, 22
century The twentieth c. will be remembered
HEALTHY LIVING, 30
cerebral they do not believe in the mind but in a c.
intestine PSYCHIATRY, 9
cesspit I see increasing evidence of people swirling
about in a human c. AIDS, 1
chair the nineteenth century was the age of the editorial c. PSYCHIATRY, 37
champagne water flowed like c. ABSTINENCE, 5
chance in our lives c. may have an astonishing influence RESEARCH, 18
chapter c. of accidents is the longest . . . in the book
ACCIDENTS, 4
charity c. offers to the poor the gains in medical skill
CHARITY, 2
The house which is not opened for c. CHARITY, 5
charlatans the c. kill. DOCTORS, 45
cheerfulness Health and c. mutually beget each other
HEALTHY LIVING, 2
chef the resurrection of a French c. HEALTHY EATING, 6
chemotherapy under the influence of modern c.
TUBERCULOSIS, 3
cherry Before the c. orchard was sold WORRY, 1
chest separating disorders of the c. from disorders of
the bowels BODY, 2
chests Men have broad and large c. SEX, 21
child A c. . . . would have no more idea of death
than a cat or a plant. DEATH, 74
all any reasonable c. can expect CONCEPTION, 4
hard travail in c. bearing BIRTH, 17
If you take away a sick C. from its Parent or Nurse
you break its Heart immediately CHILD CARE, 1
institute for the study of c. guidance CHILD CARE, 12
I would . . . stand Three times in the front of battle
than bear one c. BIRTH, 10
One stops being a c. when . . . telling one's trouble
does not make it better COUNSELLING, 3
The mother-c. relationship is paradoxical CHILD
CARE, 8
The new-born c. . . . body is more a part of himself
than surrounding objects PAIN, 13
There are only two things a c. will share willingly
CHILDREN, 3
childbearing Common morality now treats c. as an
aberration. FERTILITY, 3
childbed A man may sympathize with a woman in c.
BIRTH, 19
childbirth a matter of High Tech versus natural c.
BIRTH, 9
At the moment of c., every woman has the same
aura of isolation BIRTH, 16
childhood infancy, c., adolescence and obsolescence
AGE, 9
childishness second c. and mere oblivion SENILITY, 3
children C. do not give up their innate imagination,
curiosity, dreaminess easily CHILD CARE, 13
C., in general, are overclothed and overfed. CHILD
CARE, 4
Old men are twice c. OLD AGE, 22
our c. can give it ten or fifteen minutes EXERCISE, 7
Parents learn a lot from their c. CHILDREN, 2

copulates c. whenever she has the opportunity.
WOMEN, 16

copulation Birth, and c., and death   LIFE AND DEATH, 5

corpses does not eat c.   HEALTHY EATING, 21

couch the century of the psychiatrist's c.
PSYCHIATRY, 37

cough A c. is something that you yourself can't help
COUGHS AND COLDS, 9

coughs C. and sneezes spread diseases   COUGHS AND
COLDS, 2

were less troubled with C. when they went naked
COUGHS AND COLDS, 6

country where they're living it's peacetime, and we're all in the same c.   AIDS, 4

covetousness A physician ought to be extremely watchful against c.   DOCTORS, 31

creation Science conducts us, . . . through the whole range of c.   SCIENCE, 15

credulity natural course of the human mind is . . . from c. to scepticism   MIND, 9

creed Science . . . commits suicide when it adopts a c.   SCIENCE, 10

crippled You are not c. at all   DISABILITY, 3

crisis It may bring his distemper to a c.   DOCTORS AND
PATIENTS, 5

Nor pull a long face in a c.   DOCTORS, 8

Cross The orgasm has replaced the C.   SEX, 26

curable One is due to wax and is c.   DEAFNESS, 1

cur'd C. . . . of my disease   DOCTORS, 74

cure a c. for which there was no disease   CURES, 6

consider that the c. is discovered   CURES, 13

C. the disease and kill the patient.   CURES, 2

death is the c. of all diseases   CURES, 7

Difficult as it may be to c.   TREATMENT, 2

first you will not c. your patients   REMEDIES, 8

It is more important to c. people   DIAGNOSIS, 4

It is part of the c. to wish to be cured   CURES, 23

Nothing hinders a c. so much as frequent change of medicine   CURES, 22

People seemed to think that if he could c. an elephant he could c. anything   CURES, 8

Psychoanalysis is the disease it purports to c.
PSYCHIATRY, 34

the c. complete, he asks his fee   MEDICAL FEES, 4

The most rational c. . . . for the . . . fear of death
LIFE AND DEATH, 7

The presence of the doctor is the beginning of the c.   CURES, 21

There are maladies we must not seek to c.
REMEDIES, 16

there are only things for which man has not found a c.   CURES, 3

'There is no C. for this Disease.'   MEDICAL FEES, 5

they c. themselves   NARCOTICS, 9

We all labour against our own c.   CURES, 7

cured By opposites opposites are c.   HOMEOPATHY, 4

c. only with diet and tendering   HEALTH, 2

Groan so in perpetuity, than be c.   DEATH, 62

Only strong men are c.   NARCOTICS, 9

the only disease you don't look forward to being c. of
DEATH, 41

What can't be c.   ENDURANCE, 1

cures A good laugh and a long sleep are the best c. in the doctor's book   CURES, 18

But c. come difficult and hard   CURES, 9

he's organized these mass c.   CURES, 16

Many medicines, few c.   DRUGS, 23

Nicotinic acid c. pellagra   PREVENTIVE MEDICINE, 8

curiosity Children do not give up their innate imagination, c., dreaminess easily   CHILD CARE, 13

not for mere damnable and detestable c.
VIVISECTION, 2

The first attribute of a surgeon is an insatiable c.
SURGEONS, 18

custom A c. loathsome to the eye, hateful to the nose   SMOKING, 12

cycle this c. of good and bad days   BIORHYTHMS, 1

dad if the d. is present at the conception
CONCEPTION, 4

damn It is not true that life is one d. thing after another   LIFE, 16

damned Life is simply one d. thing after another
LIFE, 12

dark slow, sure doom falls pitiless and d.   HUMAN
CONDITION, 4

daughters D. go into analysis hating their fathers
PSYCHIATRY, 50

day Every d., in every way, I am getting better and better   PSYCHOLOGY, 3

dead If the d. talk to you, you are a spiritualist
SCHIZOPHRENIA, 3

I have been drinking it for sixty-five years and I am not d.   HEALTHY LIVING, 32

It does not then concern either the living or the d.
DEATH, 25

she was d.; but my father he kept ladling gin
CURES, 24

the living are the d. on holiday   DEATH, 46

they looked, and were, more d. than alive   FADS, 2

when you're d. it's hard to find the light switch   LIFE
AND DEATH, 2

deafness There are two kinds of d.   DEAFNESS, 1

death A child . . . would have no more idea of d. than a cat or a plant.   DEATH, 74

a disease in which d. and life are so strangely blended   TUBERCULOSIS, 1

After all, what is d.?   DEATH, 67

All interest in disease and d.   MEDICINE, 33

A long illness seems to be placed between life and d.   DEATH, 37

an intelligent man at the point of d.   DEATH, 5

Any man's d. diminishes me   DEATH, 24

A physician can sometimes parry the scythe of d.
TIME, 2

a remedy for everything except d.   REMEDIES, 5

a short and violent d.   DEATH, 45

Birth, and copulation, and d.   LIFE AND DEATH, 5

d. Will seize the doctor too   DEATH, 64

D. . . . a friend that alone can bring the peace
DEATH, 23

d. . . . can be done as easily lying down   LIFE AND
DEATH, 1

D. defies the doctor   DEATH, 55

D. has got something to be said for it: DEATH, 4

D. is a delightful hiding-place   DEATH, 31

D. is an acquired trait   DEATH, 2

D. is a punishment to some   EUTHANASIA, 6

D. is better than disease   DEATH, 39

D. is not the greatest of ills   EUTHANASIA, 7

D. is simply part of the process   DEATH, 75

d. is the cure of all diseases   CURES, 7

D. is the greatest evil   HOPE, 3

D. is the greatest kick of all   DEATH, 57

D. is the poor man's best physician   DEATH, 35

D. is the price paid by life   DEATH, 73

D. is the privilege of human nature   DEATH, 59

me . . . who is going to d.   DEATH, 40
No young man believes he shall ever d.   YOUTH, 2
Rather suffer than d.   SUFFERING, 1
seems it rich to d.   DEATH, 36
she only wants to be let d. in peace   HOSPITALS, 9
sometimes they d.   TREATMENT, 15
sooner d.   DEATH, 60
Spend all you have before you d.   HEALTHY LIVING, 26
The doctors allow one to d.   DOCTORS, 45
The human race is the only one that knows it must
d.   DEATH, 74
To d. will be an awfully big adventure   DEATH, 14
to live will be more miserable than to d.   SUICIDE, 14
We must all d.   PAIN, 18
we shall d. as usual.   DEATH, 27
Will tell me that I have to d.   DOCTORS, 8
wisdom says: 'We must d.,'   LIFE AND DEATH, 9
You will d. not because you're ill   DEATH, 50
died I d. . . . of my physician   DOCTORS, 74
dies Every moment d. a man   BIRTH, 20
He d. every day who lives a lingering life   ILLNESS, 21
He d. from his whole life   DEATH, 49
he d. in pain   LIFE AND DEATH, 10
diet A little with quiet is the only d.   HEALTHY
                                                EATING, 18
cured only with d. and tendering.   HEALTH, 2
D. away your stress   HEALTHY EATING, 17
D. cures more than the lancet   HEALTHY EATING, 1
Doctor D., Doctor Quiet and Doctor Merryman
                                                DOCTORS, 96
Food is an important part of a balanced d.   HEALTHY
                                                EATING, 12
I told my doctor I get very tired . . . on a d.
                                   HEALTHY EATING, 13
dietitians The death of all d.   HEALTHY EATING, 6
digest It's that confounded cucumber I've eat and
can't d.   INDIGESTION, 2
my stomach must just d. in its waistcoat   DRINKING, 40
To eat is human, to d. divine   INDIGESTION, 6
digestion d. is the great secret of life   DIGESTION, 2
the good or bad d. of a prime minister   DIGESTION, 3
digitalis I use d. in doses the text books say are dangerous   DRUGS, 27
dignity a paunch to give him D.   DOCTORS, 4
dimensions sickness enlarges the d. of a man's self
                                   HYPOCHONDRIA, 10
dirt he begins as d. and departs as stench   MANKIND, 32
dirtiness the other half is d.   HYGIENE, 1
discontents the family . . . source of all our d.
                                                FAMILY, 2
discover not d. new lands   RESEARCH, 19
discoverer differentiating the brilliant d. from the . . .
plodder   RESEARCH, 21
discoveries d. are usually not made by one man
alone   RESEARCH, 36
Many a man who is brooding over alleged mighty d.
                                                RESEARCH, 8
None of the great d.   RESEARCH, 14
discovery that philosophy and the knowledge of
causes led to the d.   RESEARCH, 5
Whenever science makes a d.   SCIENCE, 27
disease A bodily d., . . . whole and entire within itself   DISEASE, 7
a cure for which there was no d.   CURES, 6
a d. in which death and life are so strangely blended
                                                TUBERCULOSIS, 1
A d. known is half cured   DIAGNOSIS, 19
a d. which medicine never cured   TUBERCULOSIS, 1
All interest in d. and death   MEDICINE, 33

and so, it seems, is perfect d.   DISEASE, 8
An imaginary ailment is worse than a d.
                                   HYPOCHONDRIA, 18
a poor man for the same d. he giveth a more com-
mon name   MEDICAL FEES, 20
Choose your specialist and you choose your d.
                                                CONSULTANTS, 3
Confront d. at its first stage   DISEASE, 11
Consciousness is a d.   PSYCHOLOGY, 16
Cur'd . . . of my d.   DOCTORS, 74
Cure the d. and kill the patient.   CURES, 2
Decay and d. are often beautiful   TUBERCULOSIS, 2
Despite a lifetime of service . . . venereal d.   VENEREAL
                                                DISEASE, 1
D. can carry its ill-effects no farther than mortal
mind   CHRISTIAN SCIENCE, 2
D. creates poverty   DISEASE, 18
D. has social as well as physical, chemical, and bio-
logical causes   HOLISTIC MEDICINE, 13
D. is an experience of mortal mind   MIND AND BODY, 1
D. is an image of thought externalized   CHRISTIAN
                                                SCIENCE, 2
d. is connected only with immediate causes
                                                DISEASE, 19
D. is not of the body   DISEASE, 15
d. is the result of sin   TREATMENT, 18
D. is . . . the result of conflict between soul and
mind   DISEASE, 2
D. is very old   DISEASE, 5
D. makes men more physical   DISEASE, 9
each civilization has a pattern of d.   ENVIRONMENT, 3
Half of the secret of resistance to d. is cleanliness
                                                HYGIENE, 1
Have a chronic d. and take care of it.   LONGEVITY, 4
he does not die from the d. alone   DEATH, 49
he is a d. of the dust   MANKIND, 5
I am suffering from the particular d.   HYPOCHONDRIA, 8
I'd make health catching instead of d.   HEALTH, 9
In the nineteenth century it was a d.
                                                MASTURBATION, 6
it separates the patient from his d.   SURGEONS, 7
let us . . . eradicate d.   SCIENCE, 13
Life is a d.   LIFE, 24
Life is an incurable D.   LIFE, 7
Medicine, to produce health, has to examine d.
                                                DISEASE, 12
Natural forces are the healers of d.   HOLISTIC
                                                MEDICINE, 3
Nature cures the d.   DOCTORS, 102
Old age is a d.   OLD AGE, 38
Remedies, . . . are our great analyzers of d.
                                                REMEDIES, 13
remedies . . . suggested for a d.   REMEDIES, 6
Self-contemplation is . . . the symptom of d.
                                                PSYCHIATRY, 11
Sleep and watchfulness . . . when immoderate, constitute d.   SLEEP, 7
The aim of medicine is to prevent d.   PREVENTIVE
                                                MEDICINE, 6
the d. ceases without the use of any kind of medicine   HEALTHY LIVING, 3
The d. of an evil conscience is beyond the practice
of all the physicians   HEALTHY LIVING, 13
the d., the patient, and physician   DOCTORS AND
                                                PATIENTS, 3
the god of physic and sender of d.   MEDICINE, 55
The medicine increases the d.   DRUGS, 26
the observations of the body in health and d.
                                                NATURE, 8

the only d. you don't look forward to being cured of
                                                          DEATH, 41
the patient's personality as well as his d.   DOCTORS, 16
The prevention of d. today is one of the most important factors   PREVENTIVE MEDICINE, 5
'There is no Cure for this D.'   MEDICAL FEES, 5
the relief of d.   TREATMENT, 8
The soul is subject to health and d.   MIND AND BODY, 5
The treatment of a d. may be entirely impersonal
                                    DOCTORS AND PATIENTS, 10
tied to d.   HOLISTIC MEDICINE, 4
To prevent d., to relieve suffering and to heal the
sick   DOCTORS, 62
when the cause of d. is discovered   CURES, 13
You cure his d.   MEDICAL FEES, 3
diseases All d. run into one   OLD AGE, 19
Coughs and sneezes spread d.   COUGHS AND COLDS, 2
death is the cure of all d.   CURES, 7
D. are the tax on pleasures   DISEASE, 13
d. as isolated disturbances in a healthy body
                                                   DISEASE, 1
D. crucify the soul of man   DISEASE, 3
d. may also color the moods of civilizations
                                                  EPIDEMICS, 2
d. of their own Accord   CURES, 9
D. of the soul are more dangerous   MENTAL ILLNESS, 10
doctors themselves die of the very d. they profess to
cure   DOCTORS, 88
Extreme remedies . . . for extreme d.   REMEDIES, 11
for doctors imagine d.   ILLNESS, 16
Hungry Joe collected lists of fatal d.   HYPOCHONDRIA, 7
In acute d. it is not quite safe to prognosticate . . .
death   DIAGNOSIS, 10
Man is a museum of d.   MANKIND, 32
Medicine can only cure curable d.   MEDICINE, 14
Men worry over the great number of d.   REMEDIES, 15
new-fangled names to d.   JARGON, 19
Not even remedies can master incurable d.
                                    INCURABLE DISEASE, 2
Occupational d. are socially different from other d.
                                                  DISEASE, 17
The cure of many d. is unknown   HOLISTIC MEDICINE, 9
The deviation of man . . . seems to have proved . . .
a prolific source of d.   HEALTHY LIVING, 16
the d. which assail it   DOCTORS, 103
The d. which destroy a man   DISEASE, 14
disinfectants the best d.   ANTISEPTICS, 2
dissect Like following life through creatures you d.
                                                VIVISECTION, 6
dissections I know not, that by living d.
                                                VIVISECTION, 4
dissolve Fade far away, d.   HUMAN CONDITION, 3
distempers infectious D. must necessarily be propagated   ENVIRONMENT, 1
distinguish all there is to d. us from other animals
                                                   MANKIND, 3
diver a d. poised in albumen   PREGNANCY, 1
doctor A country d. needs more brains   DOCTORS, 71;
                                    GENERAL PRACTITIONERS, 3
A d. . . . is a patient half-cured   DOCTORS, 75
A d. is . . . licensed to make grave mistakes
                                                 DOCTORS, 49
A d. must work eighteen hours a day   DOCTORS, 25
a d. sees them as they really are.   DOCTORS, 76
a d. who has gone into lonely and discouraged
homes   DOCTORS, 50
After all, a d. is just to put your mind at rest.
                                                 DOCTORS, 69
after an interview with a d.   DOCTORS, 41

A good D. can foresee the fatal outcome of an incurable illness   INCURABLE DISEASE, 1
a good d. is one who is shrewd in diagnosis
                                                 DOCTORS, 16
a great d. kills more people than a great general
                                                 DOCTORS, 48
A man who cannot work without his hypodermic
needle is a poor d.   DRUGS, 7
a man who drinks more than his own d.   DRINKING, 2
a middle-aged d. cultivating a grey head   DOCTORS, 90
An apple a day keeps the d. away.   HEALTHY
                            EATING, 19; PREVENTIVE MEDICINE, 3
A young d. makes a full graveyard.   DOCTORS, 77
by stealing the bread denied him by his d.
                                                 DIABETES, 1
Death defies the d.   DEATH, 38
E'en dismissing the d. don't *always* succeed   CURES, 14
Even if the d. does not give you a year   INCURABLE
                                                   DISEASE, 3
Foolish the d. who despises the knowledge
                                                 DOCTORS, 37
For he was a country d., and he did not know what
it was to spare himself.   GENERAL PRACTITIONERS, 1
Fresh air impoverishes the d.   HEALTHY LIVING, 11
Give me a d. partridge-plump   DOCTORS, 8
God and the D. we alike adore   DOCTORS, 65
God is forgotten, and the D. slighted   DOCTORS, 65
He has been a d. a year now   DOCTORS, 100
he would never have died but for that vile d.
                                                 DOCTORS, 7
How does one become a good d.?   DOCTORS, 16
If you are too smart to pay the d.   MEDICAL FEES, 1
It is the duty of a d. to prolong life.   EUTHANASIA, 4
I told my d. I get very tired . . . on a diet   HEALTHY
                                                  EATING, 13
Knocked down a d.? With an ambulance?
                                                ACCIDENTS, 3
look for a d. who is hated by the best doctors.
                                                DOCTORS, 109
Make it compulsory for a d. using a brass plate
                                                 DOCTORS, 89
Nature is better than a middling d.   NATURE, 2
Never believe what a patient tells you his d. has
said.   PATIENTS, 4
No d. takes pleasure in the health even of his
friends.   DOCTORS, 56
no one ever considered the d. a gentleman
                                                 DOCTORS, 51
not even a d. can kill you   DEATH, 50
nothing more laughable than a d. who does not die
of old age   DOCTORS, 105
Our d. would never really operate unless it was necessary   MEDICAL FEES, 19
Passion, you see, can be destroyed by a d.
                                                 DOCTORS, 86
People pay the d. for his trouble   KINDNESS, 6
popular remedy often throws the scientific d. into
hysterics   REMEDIES, 7
seek out a bright young d.   DOCTORS, 109
Six men give a d. less to do than one woman
                                                   WOMEN, 22
Some d. full of phrase and fame   JARGON, 1
Than fee the d. for a nauseous draught   DRUGS, 5
The best d. in the world is the Veterinarian
                                                 DOCTORS, 81
The d. demands his fees   MEDICAL FEES, 15
The d. fainted   BIRTH, 1
The D. fared even better   CURES, 8
the d. must always be a student   TEACHING, 8

The d. occupies a seat in the front row of the stalls of the human drama   DOCTORS, 83
The D. said that Death was but A scientific fact   DEATH, 77
The d. says there is no hope   HOPE, 10
the d. takes the fee   MEDICAL FEES, 16
The essential unit of medical practice . . . seeks the advice of a d.   DOCTORS AND PATIENTS, 11
the experienced D. will take care not to aggravate the sick person's malady   INCURABLE DISEASE, 1
the inferior d. treats those who are ill   PREVENTIVE MEDICINE, 1
The most tragic thing in the world is a sick d.   DOCTORS, 87
The older a d. is and the more venerated he is   DOCTORS, 109
The presence of the d. is the beginning of the cure   CURES, 21
The real work of a d. . . . is not an affair of health centres   DOCTORS AND PATIENTS, 11
There is not a d. who desires the health of his friends   DOCTORS, 70
The relationship between d. and patient partakes of a peculiar intimacy   DOCTORS AND PATIENTS, 7
The silent d. shook his head   MEDICAL FEES, 10
The skilful d. treats those who are well   PREVENTIVE MEDICINE, 1
the successful d. was said to need three things   DOCTORS, 4
The superior d. prevents sickness   DOCTORS, 19
Three shapes a d. wears   MEDICAL FEES, 4
'What sort of d. is he?'   DOCTORS, 22
When a d. does go wrong   DOCTORS, 21
yet death will seize the d. too.   DEATH, 63
you steal a ruble from the d.   DRINKING, 35

doctoring d. either as an art or a science   DOCTORS, 5

doctors a meeting of d.   DOCTORS, 52
Call in three good d. and play bridge   COUGHS AND COLDS, 4
d. and patients   DOCTORS AND PATIENTS, 6
D. and undertakers Fear epidemics of good health   DOCTORS, 9
D. are generally dull dogs.   DOCTORS, 110
D. are just the same as lawyers   DOCTORS, 18
D. are mostly impostors.   DOCTORS, 109
D. are the most generous of men   DOCTORS, 5
d. have a front row seat   DOCTORS, 34
D., . . . know men as thoroughly as if they had made them   DOCTORS, 85
d. rob you and kill you, too   DOCTORS, 18
d. themselves die of the very diseases they profess to cure   DOCTORS, 88
for d. imagine diseases   ILLNESS, 16
I have two d.   EXERCISE, 1
I love d. and hate their medicine   DOCTORS, 108
Most of those evils . . . From d. and imagination flow.   DISEASE, 6
one cannot really have confidence in d.   DOCTORS, 32
The best d. in the world   DOCTORS, 96
The d. allow one to die   DOCTORS, 45
The d. are always changing their opinions   FADS, 3
The d. found, when she was dead   DEATH, 29
the d. know nothing   NATURE, 1
The d. were very brave about it   DOCTORS, 67
the duty of training the rising generation of d.   TEACHING, 7
The great d. all got their education off dirt pavements   MEDICAL STUDENTS, 5

There are more old drunkards than old d.   DRINKING, 15
There are only two sorts of d.   DOCTORS, 61
The trouble with d. is not that they don't know enough   DOCTORS, 20
We d. have always been a simple trusting folk.   DOCTORS, 64
when d. disagree   DOCTORS, 73
when he wears a d. cape   EVOLUTION, 22
While d. consult, the patient dies   DOCTORS, 79
Who are the greatest deceivers? The d.   DOCTORS AND PATIENTS, 13
You, as d., . . . see the human race stark naked   DOCTORS, 26
doctrine any d. . . . vouched for by . . . human beings . . . must be benighted and supersititious   SCIENCE, 12
To have admitted the truth of a d.   VACCINATION, 3
doctrines he should resist the fascination of d. and hypotheses   MEDICAL STUDENTS, 1
dogs Doctors are generally dull d.   DOCTORS, 110
dolls The fifth week, he cut out paper d.   HYPOCHONDRIA, 1
doom slow, sure d. falls pitiless and dark   HUMAN CONDITION, 4
dope Despair is better treated with hope, not d.   STRESS, 1
Science and art are only too often a superior kind of d.   NARCOTICS, 12
doses A hundred d. of happiness are not enough   DRUGS, 13
doubt faith without d. is nothing but death   FAITH, 5
douche the rattling of a thousand d. bags   CONTRACEPTION,
drained a better d. and ventilated house   HEALTHY LIVING, 27
dream waking life is a d. controlled   MENTAL ILLNESS, 40; SANITY, 4
dreaminess Children do not give up their innate imagination, curiosity, d. easily   CHILD CARE, 13
drink A taste for d., combined with gout   DRINKING, 17
D. a glass of wine after your soup   DRINKING, 35
d. may be said to be an equivocator with lechery   DRINKING, 38
d. not to elevation   HEALTHY LIVING, 12
Eat everything, d. everything and don't worry about anything   DRINKING, 43
First you take a d. . . . then the d. takes you   DRINKING, 14
I d. anything I can get my hands on   LONGEVITY, 8
One reason I don't d.   DRINKING, 1
that he has taken to d.   DRINKING, 41
We d. one another's health   DRINKING, 23
woe unto them that . . . follow strong d.   DRINKING, 7
drinking D. . . . and making love   MANKIND, 3
D. and sweating, – it's the life of a dyspeptic!   INDIGESTION, 12
I have been d. it for sixty-five years and I am not dead   HEALTHY LIVING, 32
resolve to give up smoking, d. and loving   ABSTINENCE, 1
smoking cigars and . . . d. of alcohol before, after, and . . . during   ABSTINENCE, 3
there's nothing like d.   DRINKING, 13
'Tis not the d. . . . but the excess   DRINKING, 36
drown When you go to d. yourself   SUICIDE, 21
drudgery Learn to inure yourself to d. in science   MEDICAL STUDENTS, 11
drug A d. is that substance which . . . will produce a scientific report   DRUGS, 1

E. have often been more influential than statesmen
EPIDEMICS, 2

erogenous The mind can also be an e. zone   MIND, 17;
SEX, 36

erotics e. is a perfectly respectable function of medicine   SEX, 1

error Ignorance is preferable to e.   MISTAKES, 5

errors The medical e. of one century   MISTAKES, 3

essence whether it should . . . be called the e.
DOCTORS AND PATIENTS, 7

establishment The medical e. . . . major threat to
health   MEDICAL ESTABLISHMENT, 1

ethics E. and Science need to shake hands.   MEDICAL
ETHICS, 2

the rules of medical e. were meant for young fellows
MEDICAL ETHICS, 3

events There are only three e. in a man's life
LIFE AND DEATH, 10

Everest treating the *mons Veneris* as . . . Mount E.
SEX, 12

every E. day in every way   REMEDIES, 9

evil science is . . . neither a potential for good nor for
e.   SCIENCE, 22

The greatest e. is physical pain   PAIN, 4

evils death . . . the least of all e.   DEATH, 10

Most of those e. . . . . From doctors and imagination
flow.   DISEASE, 6

the worst Of e., and excessive, overturnes All patience   PAIN, 15

evolution E. is far more important than living
EVOLUTION, 18

our views on e. would be very different EVOLUTION, 14

Some call it E.   EVOLUTION, 4

The tide of e. carries everything before it
EVOLUTION, 23

evolve Species do not e. toward perfection
EVOLUTION, 21

examination physician often hesitates to make the
necessary e.   DIAGNOSIS, 15

exception Man is an e.   MANKIND, 8

excess 'Tis not the drinking . . . but the e.
DRINKING, 36

exercise E. and temperance can preserve something
of our early strength   HEALTHY LIVING, 9

E. is bunk.   EXERCISE, 5

Fat people . . . should take their e. on an empty
stomach   EXERCISE, 6

I get my e. acting as a pallbearer   EXERCISE, 3

Patients should have rest, food, fresh air, and e.
HEALTHY LIVING, 21

The only e. I get is when I take the studs out of
one shirt   EXERCISE, 8

Thin people . . . should . . . never take e. on an
empty stomach.   EXERCISE, 6

not less than two hours a day should be devoted to
e.   EXERCISE, 7

Those who think they have not time for bodily e.
EXERCISE, 4

You've reached middle age when all you e. is caution   MIDDLE AGE, 2

existence the struggle for e.   EVOLUTION, 8

expect all any reasonable child can e.   CONCEPTION, 4

experience E. is the mother of science   RESEARCH, 32

opportunity fleeting, e. treacherous, judgment difficult   MEDICINE, 23

Reason, Observation, and E.   SCIENCE, 11

What we call e.   MISTAKES, 4

experiences the child should be allowed to meet the
real e. of life   CHILD CARE, 11

experiment a single e. can prove me wrong
RESEARCH, 12

E. alone crowns the efforts of medicine   RESEARCH, 31

experimental the e. part of medicine was first discovered   RESEARCH, 5

experimentation No amount of e. can ever prove me
right   RESEARCH, 12

expert An e. is one who knows more   CONSULTANTS, 6

explanation When there is no e., they give it a
name   JARGON, 6

explore E. thyself.   MEDITATION, 7

exquisite It is e., and it leaves one unsatisfied
SMOKING, 29

extinguishers those twin e. of science   MEDICAL FEES, 6

extreme E. remedies . . . for e. diseases   REMEDIES, 11

For e. diseases, e. methods of cure   CURES, 17

eye A custom loathsome to the e., hateful to the
nose   SMOKING, 12

A person may be indebted for a nose or an e., . . .
to a great-aunt   HEREDITY, 2

Herein are demanded the e. and the nerve
MEDITATION, 7

I have only one e.   BLINDNESS, 6

Sans teeth, sans e., sans taste   SENILITY, 3

Who formed the curious texture of the e.   EYES, 3

eyes but bein' only e. . . . my vision's limited   EYES, 1

I have a pair of e., . . . and that's just it.   EYES, 1

That youthful sparkle in his e.   EYES, 2

face till my f. falls off   OLD AGE, 13

fact the slaying of a beautiful hypothesis by an ugly f.
RESEARCH, 23

facts begin with a good body of f. and not from a
principle   RESEARCH, 9

F. are not science   SCIENCE, 5

Learn, compare, collect the f.   MEDICAL STUDENTS, 11

phantom beings loaded up with f.   SCIENCE, 26

Science is not to be regarded merely as a storehouse
of f.   SCIENCE, 7

fad Psychoanalysis is a permanent f.   PSYCHIATRY, 17

They always have some new f.   FADS, 3

faith f. without doubt is nothing but death   FAITH, 5

Nothing in life is more wonderful than f.   FAITH, 4

science and f. exclude one another.   FAITH, 6

The prayer of f. shall save the sick.   FAITH, 2

There can be no scientific dispute with respect to f.
FAITH, 6

There was a f.-healer of Deal   PAIN, 3

to those who yield it an implicit or even a partial f.
HOMEOPATHY, 6

false natural f. teeth   TEETH, 8

families All happy f. resemble one another   FAMILY, 5

family the f. . . . . source of all our discontents·
FAMILY, 2

there would never be more than *three* in a f.
BIRTH, 14

The sink is the great symbol of the bloodiness of f.
life   FAMILY, 3

fashionable every f. medical terror of the day FADS, 2

fashions I haven't the slightest idea where f. in pathology are born   FADS, 4

Medicine is like a woman who changes with the f.
FADS, 1

fast f. till he is well   HEALTHY EATING, 8

fasting F. is a medicine.   HEALTHY EATING, 11

fat A f. paunch never bred a subtle mind   OBESITY, 3

F. people . . . should take their exercise on an empty
stomach   EXERCISE, 6

I'm f. but I'm thin inside   OBESITY, 7

glands determined by the state of our ductless g. and
our viscera   MIND AND BODY, 4
Worry affects circulation, the heart and the g.
                                                    STRESS, 3
Glasgow never played the G. Empire   PSYCHIATRY, 19
glutton G., n. A person . . . committing dyspepsia
                                                INDIGESTION, 3
gluttony G. is an emotional escape HEALTHY EATING, 4
God A physician who is a lover of wisdom is the
equal to a g.   DOCTORS, 36
a pun made by G.   MANKIND, 20
At first we hail The angel; then the g.   MEDICAL
                                                 FEES, 4
G. and the Doctor we alike adore   DOCTORS, 65
G. could not be everywhere   CHILD CARE, 10
G. heals   MEDICAL FEES, 16
G. is forgotten, and the Doctor slighted   DOCTORS, 65
G.-like in our . . . breeding of . . . plants and animals
                                              EVOLUTION, 25
G. will grant an end to these too   ENDURANCE, 2
If you talk to G., you are praying   SCHIZOPHRENIA, 3
I'll die young, but it's like kissing G.   NARCOTICS, 3
I neglect G. and his angels   MEDITATION, 1
In the Nineteenth Century men lost their fear of G.
                                                  GERMS, 1
Man . . . is halfway between an ape and a g.
                                               · MANKIND, 16
The Act of G. designation   ACCIDENTS, 2
The noblest work of G.? Man   MANKIND, 33
Which is, I gather, what G. did   PSYCHOLOGY, 12
gods Whom the g. love   DEATH, 44
whom the g.-wish to destroy   MENTAL ILLNESS, 38
gold I have seen many a man turn his g. into smoke
                                                 SMOKING, 6
Silver and g. have I none   CURES, 4
the sick man hands you g. in return   MEDICAL FEES, 3
golden perhaps, the g. rule   ABSTINENCE, 10
good If . . . 'feeling g.' could decide, drunkenness
would be   DRINKING, 20
science is . . . neither a potential for g. nor for evil
                                                SCIENCE, 22
gout A taste for drink, combined with g. DRINKING, 17
Drink wine, and have the g.   GOUT, 14
For that old enemy the g.   GOUT, 11
give it another turn, and that is g.   GOUT, 2
G. is not relieved by a fine shoe   CURES, 20
G. is to the arteries what rheumatism is to the
heart.   GOUT, 12
G., n. A physician's name   GOUT, 4
if you drink wine you have the g.   GOUT, 16
I refer to g.   GOUT, 5
It is with jealousy as with the g.   GOUT, 9
Punch cures the g.   GOUT, 3
that scourge of the human race, the g.   GOUT, 8
the pleasant titillation of the g.   GOUT, 10
what is a cure for g.   GOUT, 1
when I have the g., I feel as if I was walking on my
eyeballs   GOUT, 15
we have G. for the taste   GOUT, 7
gouty My corns ache, I get g.   GOUT, 13
grave G., n. A place . . . to await the coming of the
medical student   DISSECTION, 4
graveyard A young doctor makes a full g. DOCTORS, 77
gravity the uncouth g. and supercilious self-conceit of
a physician   DOCTORS, 93
great-aunt A person may be indebted for a nose or
an eye, . . . to a g.   HEREDITY, 2
Greek prefers to describe in G.   JARGON, 2

green Anything g. that grew out of the mould
                                              HERBALISM, 4
grey a middle-aged doctor cultivating a g. head
                                               DOCTORS, 90
There is only one cure for g. hair. . . . the guillotine
                                                 CURES, 25
grief calms one's g. by recounting it   COUNSELLING, 2
it is g. that develops the powers of the mind
                                                  MIND, 14
grieve G. not that I die young   DEATH, 30
groan men sit and hear each other g.   HUMAN
                                             CONDITION, 3
grown-ups g. . . . have forgotten what it is like to be
a child   CHILDREN, 1
growth an environment equally fit for birth, g. work,
healing, and dying   HEALTHY LIVING, 14
guardian when health is restored, he is a g.
                                               DOCTORS, 1
guillotine There is only one cure for grey hair. . . .
the g.   CURES, 25
guilt fills his mind with the blackest horrors of g.
                                            HYPOCHONDRIA, 6
guinea pig consider it something monstrous to introduce under the skin of a g.   VIVISECTION, 5
gynecology A determining point in the history of g.
                                                WOMEN, 25

habits An animal psychologist is a man who pulls h.
out of rats.   PSYCHOLOGY, 1
haemorrhage retaliate upon the incompetent surgeon
is h.   SURGEONS, 16
hair A h. in the head   BALDNESS, 2
A man of forty today has nothing to worry him but
falling h.   MIDDLE AGE, 4
I think of women, it is their h.   WOMEN, 19
Man can have only a certain number of teeth, h.
and ideas   OLD AGE, 42
hand he wouldn't lay a h. on you   MEDICAL FEES, 19
'You should not bite the h. that feeds you.'   HEALTHY
                                               EATING, 25
hands don't raise your h. because I am also nearsighted   DISABILITY, 1
many brains and many h. are needed   RESEARCH, 36
handsaw I know a hawk from a h.   MENTAL ILLNESS, 44
hang I will not h. myself today   SUICIDE, 7
happened most of which had never h.   WORRY, 2
happiness Drunkenness is never anything but a substitute for h.   DRINKING, 16
Good health is an essential to h.   HEALTH, 13
h. gives us the energy   HEALTH, 1
H. is beneficial for the body   MIND, 14
happy h. families resemble each other   FAMILY, 5
Lucid intervals and h. pauses.   MENTAL ILLNESS, 1
harm the very first requirement in a Hospital that it
should do the sick no h.   HOSPITALS, 10
to help, or at least to do no h.   TREATMENT, 7
harmony So long as our souls and personalities are in
h. all is joy and peace   DISEASE, 2
harshness A sick mind cannot endure any h.   MENTAL
                                              ILLNESS, 33
hat a top h. to give him Authority   DOCTORS, 4
hawk I know a h. from a handsaw   MENTAL ILLNESS, 44
hay fever H. is the real Flower Power.   HAY FEVER, 1
heal Physician, h. thyself   DOCTORS, 11
To h. the sick   MEDICAL STUDENTS, 10
healers The best of h. is good cheer.   HEALTHY
                                               LIVING, 22
healing an environment equally fit for birth, growth
work, h., and dying   HEALTHY LIVING, 14

hips were wearing armchairs tight about the h.
                                                    OBESITY, 9
history A doctor who cannot take a good h.   CASE
                                                    HISTORY, 1
The h. of medicine does not depart from the h. of
the people.   HISTORY OF MEDICINE, 2
Homeopathy H. . . . a mingled mass of perverse ingenuity   HOMEOPATHY, 5
H. is insignificant as an act of healing
                                    HOMEOPATHY, 2
homes Healthy people are those who live in healthy
h.   HEALTHY LIVING, 14
honey water, h., and labour   REMEDIES, 20
honour Can h. set to a leg?   SURGEONS, 29
H. hath no skill in surgery   SURGEONS, 29
hope a faint h. that he will die   HUMAN NATURE, 1
Always give the patient h.   HOPE, 7
Confidence and h. do be more good than physic.
                                            HOPE, 2
He that lives upon h.   HOPE, 1
H. is necessary in every condition   HOPE, 5
H. is the physician of each misery   HOPE, 4
'Is there no h.' the sick man said   MEDICAL FEES, 10
it cuts off h.   HOPE, 3
The doctor says there is no h.   HOPE, 10
While there's life there's h.   HOPE, 8
hopefulness The first qualification for a physician is
h.   HOPE, 6
horizontally one who has ceased to grow vertically
but not h.   OBESITY, 2
hospital A h. should also have a recovery room
                                    MEDICAL FEES, 14
in a h. . . . the assumption . . . that because you
have lost your gall bladder   HOSPITALS, 5
it is against the rules of the h.   HOSPITALS, 9
Our h. organization has grown up with no plan
                                        HOSPITALS, 2
the depressing influence of general h. life
                                        HOSPITALS, 8
the h. desirable for patients with serious ailments
                                         NURSING, 6
the poor devils in the h. I am bound to take care of
                                         CHARITY, 1
the very first requirement in a H. that it should do
the sick no harm   HOSPITALS, 10
You could die very nearly as privately in a modern
h.   HOSPITALS, 1
hostages h. to fortune   FAMILY, 1
hour One h.'s sleep   SLEEP, 13
hourglass the sand in the h.   TIME, 2
human Death is the privilege of h. nature DEATH, 59
every h. creature is . . . that profound secret and
mystery   MANKIND, 9
Every man carries the entire form of h. condition
                                        MANKIND, 19
H. beings are like timid punctuation marks
                                        MANKIND, 13
H. beings, yes, but not surgeons   SURGEONS, 33
It is the h. touch after all that counts for most
                            DOCTORS AND PATIENTS, 8
my opinion of the h. race   MANKIND, 17
than it is to turn one brat into a decent h. being
                                      CHILD CARE, 12
The essence of being h.   MANKIND, 23
The h. race, . . . many of my readers   HUMAN
                                        CONDITION, 2
The h. race will be the cancer of the planet
                                        MANKIND, 15

the psychic of h. relationship between the sexes
                                            SEX, 14
To kill a h. being   EUTHANASIA, 5
You, as doctors, will be in a position to see the h.
race stark naked   DOCTORS, 26
human being A h., . . . is a whispering in the steam
pipes   MANKIND, 20
humanity H. is just a work in progress MANKIND, 35
Our h. rests upon a series of learned behaviors
                                        HEREDITY, 3
The still sad music of h.   DOCTORS, 106
the strengths and weakness of h. so completely laid
bare   DOCTORS, 57
hungry H. Joe collected lists of fatal diseases
                                     HYPOCHONDRIA, 7
hurry He sows h. and reaps indigestion
                                      INDIGESTION, 13
So who's in a h.?   DRINKING, 5
husbands that h. and wives should have children al-
ternatively   BIRTH, 14
hygiene how do drugs, h. and animal magnetism
heal?   CHRISTIAN SCIENCE, 1
h. . . . , is not much good   HYGIENE, 3
H. is the corruption of medicine by morality.
                                         HYGIENE, 5
hygienist from the point of view of the h.
                                       HOSPITALS, 3
hypochondria H. torments us not only with causeless
irritation   HYPOCHONDRIA, 13
hypochondriac ennui the h.   NEUROSIS, 5
the h. affection in men, and the hysteric in women
                                     HYPOCHONDRIA, 6
hypochondriacs H. squander large sums of time
                                     HYPOCHONDRIA, 3
hypotheses he should resist the fascination of doctrines and h.   MEDICAL STUDENTS, 1
hypothesis discard a pet h. every day before breakfast
                                        RESEARCH, 26
the slaying of a beautiful h. by an ugly fact
                                        RESEARCH, 23
hysteria I cultivate my h. with joy and terror.
                                   MENTAL ILLNESS, 2
hysteric the hypochondriac affection in men, and the
h. in women   HYPOCHONDRIA, 6
hysterical No laborious person was ever yet h.
                                         NEUROSIS, 5

id I never saw a person's i.   PSYCHOLOGY, 12
the care of the i. by the odd   PSYCHIATRY, 2
idea 'Mad' is . . . a man who is obsessed with one i.
                                   MENTAL ILLNESS, 4
ideas Man can have only a certain number of teeth,
hair and i.   OLD AGE, 42
Whenever i. fail, men invent words   JARGON, 7
idleness I. begets ennui   NEUROSIS, 5
I. is the parent of all psychology   PSYCHOLOGY, 11
ignorance for i. is never better than knowledge
                                          NATURE, 5
his chosen mode of i.   CONSULTANTS, 10
I. is preferable to error   MISTAKES, 5
opinion breeds i.   SCIENCE, 9
Why therefore fear to confess our i.? RESEARCH, 38
ignorant you can go through the wards of a hospital
and be as i.   HOSPITALS, 7
ill being i. as one of the greatest pleasures of life
                                         ILLNESS, 4
give The i. he cannot cure a name   JARGON, 1
he usually discovers that he is i. HYPOCHONDRIA, 5
I am only half there when I am i.   ILLNESS, 14

One who is i. has . . . the duty to seek medical aid
ILLNESS, 17
PHYSICIAN, n. One upon whom we set our hopes
when i.   DOCTORS, 13
the inferior doctor treats those who are i.   PREVENTIVE
MEDICINE, 1
We're all of us i. in one way or another: HEALTH, 5
When people's i., they comes to I   TREATMENT, 15
you had better be too smart to get i.   MEDICAL FEES, 1
You will die not because you're i.   DEATH, 61
illness A long i. seems to be placed between life and
death   DEATH, 37
Considering how common i. is   ILLNESS, 30
he was newly reborn from a mortal i.
CONVALESCENCE, 1
I. is in part what the world has done to a victim
ILLNESS, 18
I. isn't the only thing that spoils the appetite
HEALTHY EATING, 26
I. is the doctor to whom we pay most heed;
ILLNESS, 22
I. is the night-side of life HYPOCHONDRIA, 14; ILLNESS, 27
I. makes a man a scoundrel.   ILLNESS, 11
I. of any kind is hardly a thing to be encouraged in
others.   ILLNESS, 29
In i. the physician is a father   DOCTORS, 1
It is the part that makes the i. worth while
CONVALESCENCE, 2
No doubt fate would find it easier than I do to re-
lieve you of your i.   PSYCHIATRY, 21
Prolonged and costly i. in later years   OLD AGE, 28
sooner or later have to find time for i.   EXERCISE, 4
strange indeed that i. has not taken its place with
love   ILLNESS, 30
The doctor may also learn more about the i.
DIAGNOSIS, 9
The most important thing in i. is never to lose
heart   ILLNESS, 15
To be too conscious is an i.   ILLNESS, 6
Too much health, the cause of i.   HEALTH, 7
whether he has killed the i. or the patient   MEDICAL
FEES, 15
illnesses Most men die of their remedies, and not of
their i.   REMEDIES, 14
ills sharp remedy . . . for all i.   REMEDIES, 17
illusions dyspepsia is the apparatus of i.
INDIGESTION, 11
image make man in our own i.   MANKIND, 4
imagination a new audacity of i.   RESEARCH, 11
Children do not give up their innate i., curiosity,
dreaminess easily   CHILD CARE, 13
Most of those evils . . . From doctors and i. flow.
DISEASE, 6
imitation Man . . . is an i.   MANKIND, 24
impostors Doctors are mostly i.   DOCTORS, 109
impressed all the more i. because of the delay
DIAGNOSIS, 2
inconvenience gangrene is pain and i.   JARGON, 21
incurable A good Doctor can foresee the fatal outcome of an i. illness   INCURABLE DISEASE, 1
Not even medicine can master i. diseases.   DISEASE, 16
There are no such things as i.   CURES, 3
independent to become fully i.   CHILD CARE, 8
indigestion An i. is an excellent common-place
INDIGESTION, 8
Don't tell your friends about your i.   INDIGESTION, 7
He sows hurry and reaps i.   INDIGESTION, 13
I. is charged by God   INDIGESTION, 9

I., n. . . . frequently mistake for deep religious conviction   INDIGESTION, 4
two expressions – joy and i.   INDIGESTION, 1
indignity ultimate i. is to be given a bedpan
HOSPITALS, 6
individual the patient not only as a case but also as
an i.   DOCTORS, 16
The psychic development of the i.   PSYCHIATRY, 20
ineffable The mystic sees the i.   PSYCHIATRY, 36
inevitable ACCIDENT n. An i. occurrence   ACCIDENTS, 1
inexperience I. is what makes a young man
EXPERIENCE, 1
infancy between i. and adultery   YOUTH, 1
i., childhood, adolescence and obsolescence   AGE, 9
infants I. do not cry without some legitimate cause
CHILD CARE, 7
infection gazing into that happy future when the i.
will be banished   RESEARCH, 35
infirmity they desire but prolonged i.   OLD AGE, 7
influenza 'Ye can call it i. if ye like'   COUGHS AND
COLDS, 5
inherited infinitely fragile and never directly i.
HEREDITY, 3
inhibition Freud and his three slaves, I., Complex
and Libido   PSYCHIATRY, 33
injustice what a man still plans . . . shows the . . . i.
in his death   DEATH, 20
inner exploring Outer Space, To find the I. Man
SCIENCE, 8
insane he is pronounced i. by all smart doctors
MENTAL ILLNESS, 20
if we tried to shut up the i.   SANITY, 7
Ordinarily he is i.   MENTAL ILLNESS, 26
insanity Drunkenness is simply voluntary i.
DRINKING, 37
I. in individuals is something rare   MENTAL ILLNESS, 32
I. is hereditary   MENTAL ILLNESS, 30
I. is often the logic of an accurate mind overtaxed.
MENTAL ILLNESS, 27
Where does one go from a world of i.   MENTAL
ILLNESS, 15
insomnia every man's i. is as different from his
neighbor's   INSOMNIA, 1
I. troubles only those who can sleep any time
INSOMNIA, 2
instruction The most essential part of a student's i.
MEDICAL STUDENTS, 7
insured you cannot be i. for the accidents . . . most
likely to happen   ACCIDENTS, 2
intellect take care not to make the i. our god   MIND, 3
intelligence a story of amazing foolishness and amazing i.   HISTORY OF MEDICINE, 6
intercourse i. is . . . a social act   SEX, 9
internist An i. is someone who knows everything
CONSULTANTS, 1
interns scrub of i.   CONSULTANTS, 2
intimacy The relationship between doctor and patient
partakes of a peculiar i.   DOCTORS AND PATIENTS, 7
intoxication best of life is . . . i.   DRINKING, 11
invalid Every i. is a physician.   INVALIDS, 1
invalids the modern sympathy with i.   ILLNESS, 29
investment There is no finer i. for any community
BABIES, 1; CHILD CARE, 6
isolation At the moment of childbirth, every woman
has the same aura of i.   BIRTH, 16
itch What used to be merely an i. is now an allergy
ALLERGIES, 1

Illness is the night-side of l.   HYPOCHONDRIA, 14
Is l. worth living?   LIFE, 4
it deals with the very processes of l.   MEDICINE, 41
It is not true that l. is one damn thing after another   LIFE, 16
It is only in the microscope that our l. looks so big   LIFE, 22
its unembarrassed kindness, its insight into l.   KINDNESS, 4
Judging whether l. is or is not worth living SUICIDE, 5
L. . . . a bad dream between two awakenings.   LIFE, 19
L. as we find it is too hard for us   REMEDIES, 10
L. begins at forty   AGE, 15
L. in itself is short enough   DOCTORS, 68
L. is a disease   LIFE, 24
L. is a fatal complaint   LIFE, 11
L. is a great surprise   LIFE AND DEATH, 13
L. is an incurable Disease   LIFE, 7
L. is a partial, . . . interactive self-realization   LIFE, 2
L. . . . is a predicament.   LIFE, 20
L. is doubt   FAITH, 5
L. is made up of sobs   LIFE, 10
L. is short   MEDICINE, 23
L. is short, the art long   MEDICAL ETHICS, 4
L. is simply one damned thing after another   LIFE, 12
L. is something to do when   LIFE, 14
L. itself is but the shadow of death   LIFE AND DEATH, 4
L. itself remains a very effective therapist   PSYCHIATRY, 28
L. levels all men   LIFE AND DEATH, 14
L. protracted is protracted woe   LONGEVITY, 5
l. stands explained   MENTAL ILLNESS, 52
L., the permission to know death   LIFE AND DEATH, 2
L. to me is like boarding-house wallpaper.   LIFE, 15
L. was a funny thing   LIFE, 8
l. without it were not worth our taking   DEATH, 59
Lose a leg rather than l.   SURGEONS, 27
lot of trouble in his l.   WORRY, 2
nucleus of atoms . . . greatest secret . . . except l.   SCIENCE, 21
one must keep silent about l.   SUICIDE, 4
owe your l. to any but a regular-bred physician   DOCTORS, 91
Pain and death are a part of l.   PAIN, 7
Pain is l. – the sharper, the more evidence of l.   PAIN, 11
Progress is The law of l.   EVOLUTION, 2
The aim of l. is to live   LIFE, 17
The art of l. is the art of avoiding pain   LIFE, 13; PAIN, 10
the ascertainable laws of the science of l. are approximative   MEDICINE, 5
the child should be allowed to meet the real experiences of l.   CHILD CARE, 11
The examined l. has always been . . . confined to a privileged class.   PSYCHIATRY, 24
the paper-thin divide between l. and death   BIRTH, 9
the phenomena of l.   LIFE AND DEATH, 15
The prime goal is to alleviate suffering, and not to prolong l.   MEDICINE, 4
The purpose of human l. is to serve and to show compassion   LIFE, 23
There are only three events in a man's l.   LIFE AND DEATH, 10
to escape the l.-sentence   LIFE AND DEATH, 11
to prolong l., worry less   HEALTHY LIVING, 8
To save a man's l. against his will is . . . killing him   EUTHANASIA, 3

waking l. is a dream controlled.   MENTAL ILLNESS, 40; SANITY, 4
When he can keep l. no longer in   DEATH, 28
wherever l. is dear he is a demigod   DOCTORS, 23
While there's l. there's hope   HOPE, 8
Without health l. is not l.   HEALTH, 16
would be furious if they were suddenly restored to l.   DEATH, 48
light Are all alive with l.   BLINDNESS, 2
Doth God exact day-labour, l. deny'd   BLINDNESS, 4
like L. cures l.   HOMEOPATHY, 3
lingering He dies every day who lives a l. life   ILLNESS, 21
lips l. that touch liquor must never touch mine   ABSTINENCE, 11
liquor But l. Is quicker   DRINKING, 28
If . . . Orientals . . . drank a l.   DRINKING, 24
lips that touch l. must never touch mine   ABSTINENCE, 11
literature After twenty years one is no longer quoted in the medical l.   HISTORY OF MEDICINE, 4
live All would l. long, but none would be old   OLD AGE, 35
Do not try to l. forever.   LONGEVITY, 7
from the mouths of people who have had to l.   LIFE AND DEATH, 16
he forgets to l.   LIFE AND DEATH, 10
hence its name – liver, the thing we l. with   LIVER, 1
I eat to l.   HEALTHY EATING, 7
in order to l. in an unlivable situation   SCHIZOPHRENIA, 2
Man . . . , hath but a short time to l.   DEATH, 16
One should eat to l.   HEALTHY EATING, 15
Science says: 'We must l.,'   LIFE AND DEATH, 9
self-willed determination to l.   LIFE AND DEATH, 8
Sometimes they l.   TREATMENT, 15
They l. ill   LONGEVITY, 9
To l. is like love   LIFE, 5
to l. will be more miserable than to die   SUICIDE, 14
we l. not alone   BODY, 12
wish to l., . . . first attend your own funeral   LIFE AND DEATH, 12
You might as well l.   SUICIDE, 22
you will l. to ninety-nine   HEALTHY LIVING, 5
liver L., n. A large red organ   LIVER, 1
the positions of the l. and the heart   RESEARCH, 30
lives the stage of the disease at which he l.   LIFE, 24
You medical people will have more l. to answer for   DOCTORS, 58
living a proper way of l. be adopted   HEALTHY LIVING, 3
Evolution is far more important than l.   EVOLUTION, 18
he who lives without tobacco isn't worthy of l.   SMOKING, 20
It does not then concern either the l. or the dead   DEATH, 25
L. frugally, . . . he died early   ABSTINENCE, 2
L. is a sickness   LIFE, 6
L. well and beautifully and justly   HEALTHY LIVING, 28
the l. are the dead on holiday   DEATH, 46
logic doctoring is like l.   DOCTORS, 5
longest chapter of accidents is the l. . . . in the book   ACCIDENTS, 4
longevity L., n. Uncommon extension of the fear of death.   LONGEVITY, 1
The brain is the organ of l.   BRAIN, 10
There is no short-cut to l.   LONGEVITY, 3
looks A woman as old as she l.   AGE, 2
loss *what a l. to the state*   CHILD CARE, 5

lost not so much l. as revoked and retracted inwards
BLINDNESS, 5
love Civilized people cannot fully satisfy their sexual
instinct without l. SEX, 31
Drinking . . . and making l. MANKIND, 3
For where there is l. of man, there is also l. of the
art CHARITY, 3
L. is two minutes fifty-two seconds of squishing
noises SEX, 28
L. . . . ruined by the desire . . . legitimacy of the
children. SEX, 29
Making l. is the sovereign remedy for anguish SEX, 18
the L. that dare not speak its name HOMOSEXUALITY, 2
the most intense l. on the mother's side CHILD
CARE, 8
Without l. you will be merely skilful. OBSTETRICS, 1
Work and l. – these are the basics NEUROSIS, 14
your l. but not your thoughts CHILD CARE, 9
lucid he has l. moments when he is only stupid
MENTAL ILLNESS, 26
L. intervals and happy pauses. MENTAL ILLNESS, 1
lunatics All are l. MENTAL ILLNESS, 6
The relation between psychiatrists and other kinds of
l. PSYCHIATRY, 35
lungs don't keep using your l. LONGEVITY, 6
lyfe Long quaffing maketh a short l. DRINKING, 26

machine Man is a beautiful m. MANKIND, 18
Our body is a m. for living REMEDIES, 19
The human body is a m. BODY, 9
mad All of us are m. MENTAL ILLNESS, 5
being m. among madmen MENTAL ILLNESS, 13
Every one is more or less m. on one point. MENTAL
ILLNESS, 28
he ceased to be m. he became merely stupid
REMEDIES, 16
I am but m. north-north-west MENTAL ILLNESS, 44
Men are so necessarily m. MENTAL ILLNESS, 36
Men will always be m. MENTAL ILLNESS, 53;
PSYCHIATRY, 45
There is a pleasure sure In being m. MENTAL
ILLNESS, 14
We all are born m. MENTAL ILLNESS, 3
We want a few m. people now MENTAL ILLNESS, 46
When we remember that we are all m. MENTAL
ILLNESS, 52
Whom Fortune wishes to destroy she first makes m.
MENTAL ILLNESS, 48
M. is . . . a man who is obsessed with one idea
MENTAL ILLNESS, 4
maddest those who think they can cure them are the
m. MENTAL ILLNESS, 53
those who think they can cure them are the m. of
all PSYCHIATRY, 45
madman frightens us in a m. MENTAL ILLNESS, 21
The m. . . . has lost everything except his reason
MENTAL ILLNESS, 8
The m. thinks the rest of the world crazy. MENTAL
ILLNESS, 47
madmen The world is so full of simpletons and m.
MENTAL ILLNESS, 25
madness a dash of m. SANITY, 2
destroyed by m., starving hysterical naked MENTAL
ILLNESS, 24
every man . . . , and every woman, has a dash of m.
MENTAL ILLNESS, 18
I felt pass over me a breath of wind from the wings
of m. MENTAL ILLNESS, 2

M. and suffering can set themselves no limit.
MENTAL ILLNESS, 42
M. is part of all of us MENTAL ILLNESS, 22
M. need not be all breakdown MENTAL ILLNESS, 29
Much M. is divinest Sense MENTAL ILLNESS, 12
Our occasional m. is less wonderful MENTAL
ILLNESS, 41
Sanity is m. put to good uses MENTAL ILLNESS, 40;
SANITY, 4
The great proof of m. MENTAL ILLNESS, 31
What is m. To those who only observe MENTAL
ILLNESS, 23
What is m. MENTAL ILLNESS, 54
magic men mistook m. for medicine MEDICINE, 57
magnetism how do drugs, hygiene and animal m.
heal? CHRISTIAN SCIENCE, 1
maiden A m. at college, named Breeze WOMEN, 1
maker I am ready to meet my M. DEATH, 22
maladies Heavy thoughts bring on physical m.
HOLISTIC MEDICINE, 7
m. often have their origin there MIND AND BODY, 6
The dreary . . . tale Our mortal m. is worn and stale
HEALTH, 24
There are m. we must not seek to cure REMEDIES, 16
to call all sorts of m. people are liable to . . . , by
one name JARGON, 4
Work is the grand cure of all the m. WORK, 1
malady A reckoning up of the cause often solves the
m. CURES, 11
a single m. is more easily cured VIVISECTION, 4
Is is the m. of our age YOUTH, 3
not only the m. . . . , but also his habits when in
health HOLISTIC MEDICINE, 1
male m. and female created he them MANKIND, 4
malignant the only part of Randolph that was not m.
CANCER, 3
malingering Neurosis has an absolute genius for m.
NEUROSIS, 11
man a m. is a m. for a much longer time SEX, 2
A m. is as old as his arteries AGE, 14
A m. is not completely born BIRTH, 11
A m. of forty today has nothing to worry him but
falling hair MIDDLE AGE, 4
A m. of sixty has spent twenty years in bed LIFE, 1
a poor m. for the same disease he giveth a more
common name MEDICAL FEES, 20
A sick m. is as wayward as a child MEN, 1
a single word of it may kill a m. DOCTORS AND
PATIENTS, 4
Diseases crucify the soul of m. DISEASE, 3
Every m. carries the entire form of human condition
MANKIND, 19
Every m. has a sane spot somewhere SANITY, 6
Every m. has a wild beast within him. MANKIND, 11
he asks most insistently is about m. BODY, 5
he must view the m. in his world HOLISTIC
MEDICINE, 2
If every m. would mend a m. MEDICINE, 1
Is a m. a salvage at heart MANKIND, 2
it touches a m. that his blood is sea water
ENVIRONMENT, 4
make m. in our own image MANKIND, 4
M. always dies before he is fully born. BIRTH, 12
M. appears to be the missing link EVOLUTION, 20
M. arrives as a novice at each age of his life. AGE, 1
M., being reasonable, must get drunk DRINKING, 11
m., by possessing consciousness, is, . . . a diseased
animal PSYCHOLOGY, 16

medicine A faithful friend is the m. of life   HEALTHY
LIVING, 6
Among the arts, m., . . . must always hold the high-
est place.   MEDICINE, 8
A well chosen anthology is a complete dispensary of
m.   PREVENTIVE MEDICINE, 4
a young man entering upon the profession of m.
MEDICAL STUDENTS, 1
Better go without m.   DOCTORS, 42
By m. life may be prolonged   DEATH, 63; MEDICINE, 50
Comedy is m.   MEDICINE, 20
Common sense is in m. the master workman.
HEALING, 4; MEDICINE, 27
do not draw any distinction between food and m.
HEALTHY EATING, 14
erotics is a perfectly respectable function of m.   SEX, 1
Everything's quite different in m. nowadays
RESEARCH, 30
Experiment alone crowns the efforts of m.
RESEARCH, 31
faithful friend is the m. of life   LIFE, 3
gets well in spite of the m.   DRUGS, 15
How is it that in m. Truth is thus measured
TRUTH, 5
Hygiene is the corruption of m. by morality.
HYGIENE, 5
If the science of m. is not . . . a mere mechanical
profession   HISTORY OF MEDICINE, 1
If you want to get out of m. . . . be students all your
lives.   MEDICAL STUDENTS, 13
I love doctors and hate their m.   DOCTORS, 108
I never read a patent m. advertisement
HYPOCHONDRIA, 8
In the hands of the discoverer m. becomes a heroic
art.   MEDICINE, 16
It is a distinct art to talk m.   JARGON, 10
It is m. not scenery, for which a sick man   DRUGS, 25
It is unnecessary . . . in m. to be too clever.
DOCTORS, 40
it is useless to tell him that what he or his sick
child needs is not m.   HEALTHY LIVING, 27
I wasn't driven into m. by a social conscience
DOCTORS, 55
M. absorbs the physician's whole being   MEDICINE, 19
m. becomes a heroic art   DOCTORS, 23
M. can never abdicate the obligation to care for the
patient   MEDICINE, 54
M. can only cure curable diseases   MEDICINE, 14
M. cures the man who is fated not to die   CURES, 12
M. for the dead is too late.   MEDICINE, 45
M. is a collection of uncertain prescriptions   HEALTHY
LIVING, 20
M. is a conjectural art.   MEDICINE, 34
M. is an art   MEDICINE, 43
M. is a natural art   HISTORY OF MEDICINE, 3
M. is a noble profession   MEDICINE, 47
M. is an occupation for slaves.   MEDICINE, 48
M. is a science which hath been . . . more professed
than laboured   MEDICINE, 2
M. is as old as the human race   MEDICINE, 21
M. is a strange mixture of speculation and action.
MEDICINE, 28
M. is for the patient   MEDICINE, 37
M. is like a woman who changes with the fashions
FADS, 1
M. is not a lucrative profession.   MEDICINE, 30
M. is not only a science   MEDICINE, 41
M. is not yet liberated from the medieval idea
TREATMENT, 18

M. is the one place where all the show is stripped
of the human drama.   DOCTORS, 26
M. makes people ill   MEDICINE, 31
M. makes sick patients   ILLNESS, 16
M. may be defined as the art . . . of keeping a patient quiet   MEDICINE, 35
m. may be regarded generally as the knowledge of
the loves and desires of the body   MEDICINE, 44
m., professedly founded on observation, is as sensi-
tive to outside influences   MEDICINE, 25
M. sometimes snatches away health   MEDICINE, 40
m. still falls somewhere between trout casting and
spook writing.   MEDICINE, 22
M. . . . . the only profession that labours incessantly
MEDICINE, 7
M., to produce health, has to examine disease
DISEASE, 12
m. would be much easier   TEACHING, 3
M. would be the ideal profession   PAIN, 1
men mistook magic for m.   MEDICINE, 57
Murder with jargon where his m. fails   JARGON, 9
No families take so little m. as those of doctors
DRUGS, 12
Nothing hinders a cure so much as frequent change
of m.   CURES, 22
not the truths most commonly met with in m.
TRUTH, 4
Patience is the best m.   MEDICINE, 17
Philosophy, like m., has plenty of drugs   MEDICINE, 12
Poisons and m. are oftentimes the same substance
DRUGS, 16
Quacks in m., . . . know this, and act upon that
knowledge.   QUACKS, 4
Ready money is ready m.   HEALTH CARE, 3
Regimen is superior to m.   HEALTHY LIVING, 31
Sleep is better than m.   SLEEP, 14
Sleep's the only m. that gives ease.   SLEEP, 17
Such m. was, . . . hopelessly unscientific
TREATMENT, 13
Surely every m. is an innovation   REMEDIES, 3
that m. is not only a science   MEDICINE, 49
The aim of m. is surely not to make men virtuous
MEDICINE, 36
The aim of m. is to prevent disease   PREVENTIVE
MEDICINE, 6
The art of m. consists of amusing the patient
DOCTORS, 102
The art of m. is generally a question of time
MEDICINE, 39
The Art of M. is in need really of reasoning
MEDICINE, 11
The art of m. is my discovery.   MEDICINE, 38
The art of m. was to be properly learned only from
its practice   MEDICINE, 56
The best practitioners give to their patients the least
m.   DRUGS, 24
The care of the human mind is the most noble
branch of m.   PSYCHIATRY, 40
The foundation of the study of M.   RESEARCH, 22
The great glory of modern m.   TRUTH, 3
The history of m.   HISTORY OF MEDICINE, 6
the ideal of m. is to eliminate the need of a physi-
cian   PREVENTIVE MEDICINE, 6
The m. increases the disease   DRUGS, 26
The miserable have no other m.   HOPE, 9
the office of m. is but to tune this curious harp of
man's body   MEDICINE, 3
The only sure foundations of m.   MEDICINE, 26

Pain of m. is worse than pain of body   MENTAL
                                                    ILLNESS, 49
Physicians must discover the weaknesses of the
human m.   DIAGNOSIS, 6
So long as the body is affected through the m.
                                                    HOMEOPATHY, 6
the best medicines for an afflicted m.   WORK, 3
The care of the human m. is the most noble branch
of medicine   PSYCHIATRY, 40
The conscious m. may be compared to a fountain
                                                    MIND, 5
The highest function of M.   MIND, 11
The m. can also be an erogenous zone   MIND, 17;
                                                    SEX, 36
The m. grows sicker than the body MENTAL ILLNESS, 35
The m. has great influence over the body   MIND AND
                                                    BODY, 6
The m. is an iceberg   MIND, 4
The m. like a sick body can be healed   MIND, 12
the m. must sweat a poison   BRAIN, 7
the most abhorrent is body without m.   SENILITY, 2
The pendulum of the m.   MIND, 10
the prison of our m.   MIND, 15
The psychiatrist is the obstetrician of the m.
                                                    PSYCHIATRY, 3
The remarkable thing about the human m.   MIND, 7
they do not believe in the m. but in a cerebral intestine   PSYCHIATRY, 9
unless your m. is in a splint   DISABILITY, 3
we consider as nothing the rape of the human m.
                                                    MIND AND BODY, 3
Well in body But sick in m.   HOLISTIC MEDICINE, 10
minds All things can corrupt perverted m.   MENTAL
                                                    ILLNESS, 34
great m. in the commonplace   MIND, 8
Little m. are interested in the extraordinary   MIND, 8
many open m. should be closed for repairs   MIND, 1
M. like bodies, will often fall into a pimpled, ill-
conditioned state   MIND, 2
Old age puts more wrinkles in our m. than on our
faces.   OLD AGE, 32
Our m. are lazier than our bodies   MIND AND BODY, 7
the m. of the people are closed   HOLISTIC MEDICINE, 4
to lead ignorant and prejudic'd m.   RESEARCH, 25
When people will not weed their own m.   MIND, 16
mirth to fence against the infirmities of ill health . . .
by m.   HEALTHY LIVING, 29
miscarriage procure thee m.   ABORTION, 6
they induce herbs . . . to cause m.   ABORTION, 1
miseries makes men's m. of alarming brevity CURES, 10
misery if we succeed in transforming your hysterical
m. into common unhappiness   PSYCHIATRY, 21
Thou art so full of m.   SUICIDE, 29
mistake A m. in other professions is tolerable
                                        MISTAKES, 6
Man is Nature's sole m.   MANKIND, 12
mistakes A doctor is . . . licensed to make grave m.
                                        DOCTORS, 49
a dreadful list of ghastly m.   MISTAKES, 4
moan That is not paid with m.   PAIN, 21
modern So it was all m. and scientific and well-arranged.   HOSPITALS, 1
money a blessing that m. cannot buy   HEALTH, 22
If he didn't need the m.   MEDICAL FEES, 19
I only take m. from sick people.   HYPOCHONDRIA, 2
the soul of a m. changer   MEDICAL FEES, 7
monkey I could never look long upon a M., without
very Mortifying Reflections.   EVOLUTION, 5

monkeys we are descended not only from m. but
from monks.   EVOLUTION, 16
mons treating the m. Veneris as . . . Mount Everest
                                        SEX, 12
month if he hesitates about a m.   INCURABLE DISEASE, 3
moon The m. is nothing But a circumambulating
aphrodisiac   FERTILITY, 1
morality Hygiene is the corruption of medicine by m.
                                        HYGIENE, 5
there is such a thing as physical m.   HEALTH, 20
more Specialist – A man who knows m. and m.
about less and less   CONSULTANTS, 11
morphia have yourself squirted full of m.   DEATH, 34
mortal Her last disorder m.   DEATH, 29
'Remember that I too am m.'   DOCTORS, 89
mortality Reduce the m. rate, consult doctors   CHILD
                                        CARE, 5
mother A smart m. makes often a better diagnosis
                                        DIAGNOSIS, 3
I wished to be near my m.   BIRTH, 12
the most intense love on the m.'s side CHILD CARE, 8
The m.-child relationship is paradoxical CHILD CARE, 8
motherhood wifehood and m. are but incidental relations   WOMEN, 27
mother love M., . . . is a highly respected and much
publicized emotion   WOMEN, 7
mothers therefore he made m.   CHILD CARE, 10
unfair not only to the m. and ancestors HISTORY OF
                                        MEDICINE, 5
mould Anything green that grew out of the m.
                                        HERBALISM, 4
mouth need not look in your m.   AGE, 12
multiply be fruitful and m.   MANKIND, 4
The command 'Be fruitful and m.'   CONTRACEPTION, 4
muscles a network of nerves and m. and tissues in-
flamed'by disease   ANATOMY, 5
music The still sad m. of humanity   DOCTORS, 106
mutton people who do not object to eating a m.
chop   VIVISECTION, 5
mystic The m. sees the ineffable   PSYCHIATRY, 36
mystical to stimulate the m. faculties of human nature   DRINKING, 21
naked The exception is a n. ape   MANKIND, 21
name to call all sorts of maladies . . . by one n.
                                        JARGON, 4
When there is no explanation, they give it a n.
                                        JARGON, 6
names new-fangled n. to diseases   JARGON, 19
There is no counting the n., that surgeons and
anatomists give   JARGON, 17
narcotic The amount of n. you use is inversely pro-
portional to your skill   DRUGS, 7
narcotics Two great European n.   DRINKING, 29
natural n. false teeth   TEETH, 8
N. Selection   EVOLUTION, 9
nature go into partnership with n.   NATURE, 1
I have always respected suicide as a regulator of n.
                                        SUICIDE, 19
I watched what method N. might take   NATURE, 15
Man is N.'s sole mistake   MANKIND, 12
N. can do more than physicians   NATURE, 3
N. has always had more power than education
                                        NATURE, 16
N. heals, under the auspices of the medical profes-
sion.   NATURE, 4
N., in medical language   TREATMENT, 8
N. is a benevolent old hypocrite   NATURE, 10
n. is a conjugation of the verb to eat NATURE, 12

N. is better than a middling doctor NATURE, 2
N. puts upon no man an unbearable burden SUICIDE, 19
N., time, and patience are the three great physicians DOCTORS, 78; MEDICINE, 9
Of all the soft, delicious functions of n. this is the chiefest SLEEP, 18
Oh, the powers of n. NATURE, 1
Our foster nurse of n. is repose SLEEP, 15
The art of healing comes from n. NATURE, 13
the disease is cured by n. NATURE, 7
the encroachment of n. NATURE, 9
The physician is N.'s assistant. DOCTORS, 28
The physician is only the servant of n. NATURE, 14
the physician must start from n. NATURE, 13
the surgeon be sometimes tempted to supplant in-stead of aiding N. SURGEONS, 23
Though you drive away N. NATURE, 11
until n. kills him or cures him. MEDICINE, 35
We must turn to n. itself NATURE, 8
Whatever N. has in store for mankind NATURE, 5
near I wished to be n. my mother BIRTH, 21
nearsighted don't raise your hands because I am also n. DISABILITY, 1
nerve called a n. specialist because it sounds better PSYCHIATRY, 49
Herein are demanded the eye and the n. MEDITATION, 7
nerves a network of n. and muscles and tissues in-flamed by disease ANATOMY, 5
grates on our n. NEUROSIS, 7
nervous winding up its n. and intellectual system to the utmost point SUICIDE, 12
you're being attacked by the n. system NERVOUS SYSTEM, 1
nettles apt to be overrun with n. MIND, 16
neurasthenia he is put there with the diagnosis of n. PSYCHIATRY, 29
neurosis
by accepting the universal n. he is spared . . . a per-sonal n. NEUROSIS, 3
Modern n. began with the discoveries of Copernicus NEUROSIS, 8
N. has an absolute genius for malingering NEUROSIS, 11
N. is always a substitute for legitimate suffering NEUROSIS, 6
N. is the way of avoiding non-being NEUROSIS, 15
the Age of Anxiety, the age of the n. NEUROSIS, 7
the secret of n. is to be found in the family battle of wills NEUROSIS, 10
Without them there is n. NEUROSIS, 14
neurotic A n. is the man who builds a castle in the air. PSYCHIATRY, 46
he suffered . . . the n. ills of an entire generation NEUROSIS, 4
N. means he is not as sensible as I am NEUROSIS, 9
Psychiatrists classify a person as n. PSYCHIATRY, 43
the n. person knows that two and two make four NEUROSIS, 1
neurotics A mistake which is commonly made about n. NEUROSIS, 2
Everything great in the world comes from n. NEUROSIS, 12
The 'sensibility' claimed by n. NEUROSIS, 13
nicotinic N. acid cures pellagra PREVENTIVE MEDICINE, 8
night calm passage . . . across many a bad n. SUICIDE, 20
Do not go gentle into that good n. DEATH, 72

Job was never on n. duty. NURSING, 8
noise A loud n. at one end BABIES, 3
nomenclature even the learned ignorance of a n. JARGON, 14
nose A custom loathsome to the eye, hateful to the n. SMOKING, 12
A person may be indebted for a n. . . . to a great-aunt HEREDITY, 2
nourisher Chief n. in life's feast SLEEP, 16
novice Man arrives as a n. at each age of his life. AGE, 1
nurse a good n. is of more importance than a physi-cian NURSING, 4
from the point of view of the hygienist . . . and the n. HOSPITALS, 3
If ye had a good n. NURSING, 2
It's better to be sick than n. the sick NURSING, 3
Our foster n. of nature is repose SLEEP, 15
Talk of the patience of Job, said a Hospital n. NURSING, 8
That person alone is fit to n. or to attend the bed-side of a patient NURSING, 9
The trained n. has become one of the great bless-ings of humanity NURSING, 7
The trained n. has given nursing the human . . . touch NURSING, 6
nurses a giggle of n. CONSULTANTS, 2
nursing n. means vexation of the mind NURSING, 3

obesity O. is a mental state OBESITY, 6
oblivion second childishness and mere o. SENILITY, 3
observation medicine, professedly founded on o. MEDICINE, 25
Reason, O., and Experience SCIENCE, 11
the gift of keen o. MEDICINE, 32
obsolescence infancy, childhood, adolescence and o. AGE, 9
obstetrician The psychiatrist is the o. of the mind PSYCHIATRY, 3
obvious the analysis of the o. RESEARCH, 40
occupations There are worse o. in the world than feeling a woman's pulse DOCTORS, 94
octopus dear o. from whose tentacles we never quite escape FAMILY, 4
odd the care of the id by the o. PSYCHIATRY, 2
ointment Time cures the sick man, not the o. TIME, 3
old All would live long, but none would be o. OLD AGE, 35
An o. man looks permanent OLD AGE, 9
Dying while young is a boon in o. age OLD AGE, 44
first sign of o. age OLD AGE, 24
Forty is the o. age of youth OLD AGE, 20
Growing o. is a bad habit OLD AGE, 31
If you want to be a dear o. lady at seventy OLD AGE, 37
in these qualities o. age is usually not only not poorer OLD AGE, 17
No skill or art is needed to grow o. OLD AGE, 21
o. age a regret AGE, 4
O. age is a disease OLD AGE, 38
o. age is always fifteen years older than I am. OLD AGE, 8
O. age is an island surrounded by death OLD AGE, 33
O. age puts more wrinkles in our minds than on our faces. OLD AGE, 32
O. men are twice children OLD AGE, 22
Physicians, . . . , are best when they are o. DOCTORS, 27

so few who can grow o. with a good grace   OLD
AGE, 41
the misery of an o. man is interesting to nobody
OLD AGE, 25
the o. have reminiscences   MEMORY, 2
The principal objection to o. age   OLD AGE, 3
Tidy the o. into tall flats.   OLD AGE, 10
We grow o. more through indolence   OLD AGE, 16
What makes o. age hard to bear   OLD AGE, 30
When men desire o. age   OLD AGE, 7
Why does he die of o. age?   BODY, 5
You are getting o. when the gleam in your eyes   OLD
AGE, 4
you grow o. beautifully.   OLD AGE, 29
'You have lived to be an o. man,'   DOCTORS AND
PATIENTS, 9
older As you get o. . . . more boring   OLD AGE, 36
one is to grow o., the other not   OLD AGE, 1
to go on getting o.   TREATMENT, 1
on they get o., then they get *honour*   DOCTORS, 82
Onan O. knew that the seed should not be his
MASTURBATION, 3
one-eyed the O. Man is King   BLINDNESS, 10
oneself the only person with whom one dares to talk
continually of o.   MEDICAL FEES, 11
operate Our doctor would never really o. unless it
was necessary   MEDICAL FEES, 19
to o. upon Queen Victoria   SURGEONS, 22
operating Speed in o. should be the achievement
SURGEONS, 20
The most important person in the o. theatre is the
patient   SURGEONS, 19
operation Before undergoing a surgical o.   SURGEONS, 15
Exploratory o.: a remunerative reconnaissance.
MEDICAL FEES, 2
I never say of an o. that it is without danger.
SURGEONS, 5
I see but as one sees after an o.   BLINDNESS, 1
The feasibility of an o.   SURGEONS, 6
The o. wasn't bad   SURGEONS, 34
The o. was successful – but the patient died
SURGEONS, 2
when an o. is once performed   SURGEONS, 31
operations I am of the opinion my o. rather kept
down my practice   SURGEONS, 9
the king of all topics is o.   SURGEONS, 8
ophthalmologists eyeful of o.;   CONSULTANTS, 2
opiate O. An unlocked door in the prison of Identity
NARCOTICS, 2
opinion he is . . . Now but a climate of o.
PSYCHIATRY, 5
o. breeds ignorance   SCIENCE, 9
opinions The doctors are always changing their o.
FADS, 3
opium O. gives and takes away   NARCOTICS, 7
O. is pleasing to Turks   NARCOTICS, 4
O. . . . the Creator himself seems to prescribe
NARCOTICS, 11
subtle, and mighty o.   NARCOTICS, 6
To tell the story of Coleridge without the o.
NARCOTICS, 14
opportunity o. fleeting, experience treacherous, judgment difficult   MEDICINE, 23
opposites By o. o. are cured   HOMEOPATHY, 4
oppressed The o. speak a million tongues   MENTAL
ILLNESS, 50
optimism O.: A kind of heart stimulant   FAITH, 3
The place where o. most flourishes is the lunatic
asylum   MENTAL ILLNESS, 17

optimistic O. lies   MEDICINE, 51
orchard Before the cherry o. was sold   WORRY, 1
organ an amplification of one o.   MEDICINE, 15
A physician is obligated to consider more than a
diseased o.   HOLISTIC MEDICINE, 2
The only bodily o. which is really regarded as inferior   WOMEN, 12
organs To be solemn about the o. of generation
SEX, 15
orgasm One o. in the bush   MASTURBATION, 5
The o. has replaced the Cross   SEX, 26
Orientals If . . . O. . . . drank a liquor which . . .
made them vomit   DRINKING, 24
origin the indelible stamp of his lowly o.   EVOLUTION, 6
outer exploring O. Space, To find the Inner Man.
SCIENCE, 8
outlive do not o. yourself   HEALTHY LIVING, 26
overrun apt to be o. with nettles   MIND, 16
ovule Man is developed from an o.   CONCEPTION, 1
ovules differs in no respect from the o. of other animals   CONCEPTION, 1

pain But p. is perfect miserie   PAIN, 15
For we are born in others' p.   PAIN, 21
gangrene is p. and inconvenience   JARGON, 21
He that is uneasy at every little p.   HYPOCHONDRIA, 12
hour of p. is as long   PAIN, 17
if it did not involve giving p.   PAIN, 1
it entails too much p.   REMEDIES, 10
it is only by degrees, through p., that he under-
stands the . . . body   PAIN, 13
It would be a great thing to understand P.   PAIN, 12
Man endures p. as an undeserved punishment   PAIN, 2
Much of your p. is self-chosen.   PAIN, 8
my considerable daily allotment of p.   INDIGESTION, 5
Neither poverty nor p. is accumulable.   PAIN, 5
P. and death are a part of life   PAIN, 7
P. – has an Element of Blank   PAIN, 6
P. is a more terrible lord of mankind than even
death himself   PAIN, 18
P. is life – the sharper, the more evidence of life.
PAIN, 11
p. isn't real   PAIN, 3
P. is the correlative of some species of wrong
PAIN, 20
P. of mind is worse than pain of body   MENTAL
ILLNESS, 49
P. was my portion   DEATH, 7
p. we obey   ILLNESS, 22
P. with the thousand teeth.   PAIN, 23
Remember that p. has this most excellent quality
PAIN, 19
The art of life is the art of avoiding p.   LIFE, 13;
PAIN, 10
The first cry of p. . . . was the first call for a physi-
cian   HISTORY OF MEDICINE, 3
The greatest evil is physical p.   PAIN, 4
the momentary intoxication with p.   MENTAL ILLNESS, 7
Time heals old p.   PAIN, 9
To cease upon the midnight with no p.   DEATH, 36
painful the one is as p. as the other   BIRTH, 2
pains suffering her p. in his own proper person and
character   BIRTH, 19
With what shift and p. we come into the World
DEATH, 17
paralyse p. it by encumbering it with remedies
REMEDIES, 19
paralysis p. is nervousness   JARGON, 21
paranoid Just because you're p.   PSYCHIATRY, 1

parasite The sick man is a p. of society   INVALIDS, 2
parents From birth to age eighteen, a girl needs good
p.   AGE, 16
P. are the last people on earth   CHILD CARE, 3
P. learn a lot from their children   CHILDREN, 2
parts there are no spare p.   TRANSPLANTS, 1
parturates p. once a year   WOMEN, 16
parturition P. is a physiological process   BIRTH, 7
pass To p. away ere life hath lost its brightness
DEATH, 30
passage a fair and easie p. for it to go out   DEATH, 28
calm p. . . . across many a bad night   SUICIDE, 20
passion Asthma is a disease that has practically the
same symptoms as p.   ASTHMA, 1
past half of you belongs to the p.   MIDDLE AGE, 3
patent The people – could you p. the sun?   POLIO, 1
pathologist an ulcer is wonderful to a p.   PATHOLOGY, 1
A p. is someone who knows everything
CONSULTANTS, 1
pathologists there were p. present   DOCTORS, 52
pathology I haven't the slightest idea where fashions
in p. are born   FADS, 4
patience Nature, time, and p. are the three great
physicians   DOCTORS, 78; MEDICINE, 9
P. is the best medicine   MEDICINE, 17
Talk of the p. of Job, said a Hospital nurse   NURSING, 8
the worst Of evils, and excessive, overturnes All p.
PAIN, 15
patient A doctor . . . is a p. half-cured   DOCTORS, 75
An unruly p. makes a harsh physician   DOCTORS, 97
A physician who treats himself has a fool for a p.
DOCTORS, 63
Before you tell the 'truth' to the p.   TRUTH, 1
cure their p. and lose their fee   MEDICAL FEES, 18
First, the p.   PATIENTS, 5
from the point of view of the p.   HOSPITALS, 3
from the way the p. tells the story than from the
story itself   DIAGNOSIS, 9
He turns into a life-long p.   HEALTH CARE, 1
if the p. can keep awake, surely you can
ANAESTHESIA, 4
INDIGESTION, n. A disease which the p. and his
friends frequently mistake for deep religious convic-
tion   INDIGESTION, 4
It is the p. rather than the case which requires
treatment   TREATMENT, 17
It is too bad that we cannot cut the p. in half
RESEARCH, 34
it separates the p. from his disease   SURGEONS, 7
Keep up the spirits of your p.   TREATMENT, 16
Medicine can never abdicate the obligation to care
for the p.   MEDICINE, 54
Medicine is for the p.   MEDICINE, 37
Never believe what a p. tells you his doctor has
said.   PATIENTS, 4
Once in a while you will have a p. of sense
PATIENTS, 2
the analyst should pay the p.   PSYCHIATRY, 44
the care of a p. must be completely personal
DOCTORS AND PATIENTS, 10
The consultant's first obligation is to the p.
CONSULTANTS, 9
the disease, the p., and physician   DOCTORS AND
PATIENTS, 3
The most important person in the operating theatre
is the p.   SURGEONS, 19
The p. has been so completely taken to pieces
PATIENTS, 6
The p. lingers and by inches dies   DOCTORS, 30

The p. must co-operate with the physician in com-
bating the disease   DOCTORS AND PATIENTS, 3
The p. never dies   SKIN, 1
the p. not only as a case but also as an individual
DOCTORS, 16
Therein the p. Must minister to himself.   MENTAL
ILLNESS, 45
The relationship between doctor and p. partakes of
a peculiar intimacy   DOCTORS AND PATIENTS, 7
The safest thing for a p.   TEACHING, 8
to secure the co-operation of the p.   MEDICAL ETHICS, 4
We first do everything for the p.   PATIENTS, 5
What I call a good p.   PATIENTS, 3
patients A clinician shall deal honestly with p.
MEDICAL ETHICS, 1
all of his p. being willing to steal   MEDICAL FEES, 12
doctors and p.   DOCTORS AND PATIENTS, 6
He never sees his p.   CURES, 16
his p. should be his book   DOCTORS, 66
my p. would have recovered without the use of
physic   TREATMENT, 11
P. consult so-called authorities   CONSULTANTS, 4
p. who don't eat   ANOREXIA, 1
Private p., if they do not like me, can go elsewhere
CHARITY, 1
Psychoanalysts are not occupied with the minds of
their p.   PSYCHIATRY, 9
Some p., though conscious that their condition is
perilous   DOCTORS, 38
The best practitioners give to their p. the least medicine   DRUGS, 24
the faults of the p.   DRUGS, 10
the greatest fools? The p.   DOCTORS AND PATIENTS, 13
the p. personality as well as his disease   DOCTORS, 16
There are some p. whom we cannot help
TREATMENT, 3
Too often a sister puts all her p. back to bed
NURSING, 1
you will have no p. to cure.   REMEDIES, 8
paunch a p. to give him Dignity   DOCTORS, 4
peace So long as our souls and personalities are in
harmony all is joy and p.   DISEASE, 2
you buy a pill and buy p.   DRUGS, 17
peacetime where they're living it's p. and we're all in
the same country   AIDS, 4
pediatricians P. eat because children don't
CONSULTANTS, 13
pelican A fashionable surgeon like a p.   MEDICAL FEES, 9
pellagra Nicotinic acid cures p.   PREVENTIVE MEDICINE, 8
penis he also has the biggest p.   MEN, 2
people The p. – could you patent the sun?   POLIO, 1
perfect A cigarette is . . . a p. pleasure   SMOKING, 29
perfection one does not seek p.   MANKIND, 23
Species do not evolve toward p.   EVOLUTION, 21
performance desire should . . . outlive p.   SEX, 32
it takes away the p.   DRINKING, 38
period Never neglect the history of a missed menstrual p.   CONCEPTION, 3
perish Cause thy fruit to p.   ABORTION, 6
person A p. may be indebted for a nose or an eye,
. . . to a great-aunt   HEREDITY, 2
personality the patient's p. as well as his disease
DOCTORS, 16
perversion that melancholy sexual p. known as continence   ABSTINENCE, 6
pervert Once: a philosopher; twice: a p.!   SEX, 34
pharmacopoeia Water, air, and cleanliness are the
chief articles in my p.   HEALTHY LIVING, 20

Take care not to fancy that you are p.   MEDICAL
                                               STUDENTS, 14
Temperance and labour are the two real p. of man:
                                                    WORK, 4
that p. are the class of people who kill other men
                                                DOCTORS, 84
The crowd of p. has killed me   DOCTORS, 33
The disease of an evil conscience is beyond the
practice of all the p.   HEALTHY LIVING, 13
The most dangerous p.   DOCTORS, 59
the old p. have supplied the undertaker DISSECTION, 3
The p. are here, too.   DOCTORS, 52
The p. are the natural attorneys of the poor
                                               DOCTORS, 101
The p. best remedy is *Tincture of Time!*   TIME, 4
the p. separate the soul from the body   HOLISTIC
                                               MEDICINE, 9
the p. with their art, know . . . how to make it still
shorter   DOCTORS, 68
the p. words will be received with just that much
more attention   DIAGNOSIS, 2
The sick man is the garden of the p.   DOCTORS AND
                                               PATIENTS, 12
Three remedies of the p. of Myddfai   REMEDIES, 20
two p. cure you of the medicine   DOCTORS, 3
physicist The great p. Lavoisier, who knew better
than any peasant   SCIENCE, 1
physics The content of p. is the concern   SCIENCE, 4
physiology an important part of reproductive p.   SEX, 1
pie A word of kindness is better than a fat p.
                                              KINDNESS, 5
piles p. to give him an Anxious Expression
                                                DOCTORS, 4
pill buy a p. and buy peace with it   MEDICINE, 29
Protestant women may take the P. CONTRACEPTION, 10
you buy a p. and buy peace   DRUGS, 17
pillow no-sooner-have-I-touched-the-p. people
                                                  SLEEP, 11
pills It is an age of p.   DRUGS, 19
I will lift up mine eyes unto the p.   DRUGS, 19
One of the most successful physicians . . . has . . .
used more bread p.   DRUGS, 14
piping Helpless, naked, p. loud   BIRTH, 6
pitiless slow, sure doom falls p. and dark   HUMAN
                                               CONDITION, 4
planet The human race will be the cancer of the p.
                                               MANKIND, 15
plans what a man still p. . . . shows the . . . injustice
in his death   DEATH, 20
plants tend to make us forget the medicinal value of
p.   HERBALISM, 3
pleasant P. words are as an honeycomb, sweet to the
soul   KINDNESS, 1
pleasure For physical p. I'd sooner go to the dentist
any day.   SEX, 35
The p. is momentary, the position ridiculous   SEX, 7
There is a p. sure In being mad MENTAL ILLNESS, 14
what p. . . . they have in taking their roguish tobacco   SMOKING, 15
pleasures being ill as one of the greatest p. of life
                                                 ILLNESS, 4
Diseases are the tax on p.   DISEASE, 13
interfering with the p. of others   ABSTINENCE, 9
plumbing an ingenious assembly of portable p.
                                               MANKIND, 20
pneumonia When a man lacks mental balance in p.
                                          MENTAL ILLNESS, 20
poems The few bad p. . . . created during abstinence
                                              ABSTINENCE, 7

poets The p. and philosophers . . . have discovered
the unconscious   PSYCHIATRY, 22
poison it is always easy to p. and to kill TREATMENT, 2
Neither will I administer a p. to anybody   MEDICAL
                                                ETHICS, 5
Psychology is as unnecessary as directions for using
p.   PSYCHOLOGY, 8
The treatment with p. medicines comes from the
West.   TREATMENT, 10
wounds and abscesses no longer p. the atmosphere
                                              ANTISEPTICS, 1
poisons P. and medicine are oftentimes the same substance   DRUGS, 16
The p. are our principal medicines   DRUGS, 6
two p. are more efficacious than one   DRUGS, 3
pole Beloved from p. to p.   SLEEP, 2
policemen how young the p. look   OLD AGE, 24
pomp I will make the p. of emperors ridiculous
                                                 HEALTH, 6
poor choosing to store her money in the stomachs of
the p.   CHARITY, 4
health! the blessing of the rich! the riches of the p.
                                                HEALTH, 10
If a patient is p. he is committed . . . as 'psychotic'
                                              PSYCHIATRY, 29
pays equal attention to the rich and the p.
                                               DOCTORS, 103
the p. devils in the hospital I am bound to take
care of   CHARITY, 1
population when the p. of the world consisted of two
people   CONTRACEPTION, 4
position The pleasure is momentary, the p. ridiculous
                                                    SEX, 7
post-mortem In the p. room we witness the final result of disease   POST-MORTEM, 1
poverty Disease creates p.   DISEASE, 18
power Hay fever is the real Flower P.   HAY FEVER, 1
powerless Brief and p.   HUMAN CONDITION, 4
practice P. should always be based upon a sound
knowledge of theory   THEORY, 3
Tact is a valuable attribute in gaining p.   DOCTORS
                                             AND PATIENTS, 1
The essential unit of medical p. is   DOCTORS AND
                                               PATIENTS, 11
practitioner A general p. can no more become a specialist   GENERAL PRACTITIONERS, 2
practitioners this is full of danger if its p. are not
perfect   MISTAKES, 6
pregnancy quite lawful for a Catholic woman to
avoid p. by . . . mathematics   CONTRACEPTION, 6
pregnant in women nine out of ten abdominal swellings are the p. uterus   PREGNANCY, 3
prejudice If you are hidebound with p.   HOSPITALS, 7
prejudices my p. swell like varicose veins   GOUT, 13
prescribed the taking of things p.   DRUGS, 10
preserves What destroys one man p. another
                                                  CURES, 15
prevent not knowing how to p. them
                                           CONTRACEPTION, 8
preventing a means of p. it.   PREVENTIVE MEDICINE, 7
prevention P. of disease must become the goal of every physician.   PREVENTIVE MEDICINE, 9
The p. of disease today is one of the most important
factors   PREVENTIVE MEDICINE, 5
preventive one ultimate and effectual p. . . . is death
                                   PREVENTIVE MEDICINE, 2
the promotion of it is a branch of p. medicine
                                               LONGEVITY, 3
prevents a beefsteak p. it   PREVENTIVE MEDICINE, 8

priest A p. sees people at their best   DOCTORS, 76
taking a place beside the physician and the p.
                                                   NURSING, 7
principle begin with a good body of facts and not
from a p.   RESEARCH, 9
prison a sick, its p.   BODY, 1
the p. of our mind   MIND, 15
privacy at least 45 minutes of undisturbed p.
                                                   HOSPITALS, 11
private He was meddling too much in my p. life
                                                   PSYCHIATRY, 48
P. practice and marriage   MEDICAL FEES, 6
The human body is p. property.   RESEARCH, 29
procreation Abortion . . . an appalling trivialization of
. . . p.   ABORTION, 2
proctologists pile of p.   CONSULTANTS, 2
professed Medicine is a science which hath been . . .
more p. than laboured   MEDICINE, 2
professor A p. is a gentleman who has a different
opinion.   TEACHING, 2
professors If there weren't so many p.   TEACHING, 3
Progress P. is The law of life   EVOLUTION, 2
progression the labour having been . . . rather in a
circle than in p.   MEDICINE, 2
proof The great p. of madness   MENTAL ILLNESS, 31
propagated wished that mankind were p. like trees
                                                   SEX, 16
propagation Women exist . . . solely for the p. of the
species   WOMEN, 24
Protestant P. women may take the Pill
                                           CONTRACEPTION, 10
psyche the human p. lives in indissoluble union with
the body   PSYCHOLOGY, 7
psychedelics discovery of p. one of the three major
scientific break-throughs   NARCOTICS, 13
psychiatric a person who so obviously needs p. attention   PSYCHIATRY, 14
psychiatrist And a p. is the man who collects the
rent.   PSYCHIATRY, 46
A p. is a man who goes to the Folies-Bergère
                                           PSYCHIATRY, 42
A p. is someone who knows nothing   CONSULTANTS, 1
I know that each conversation with a p.
                                           PSYCHIATRY, 4
No man is a hero to his wife's p.   PSYCHIATRY, 10
One should only see a p. out of boredom.
                                           PSYCHIATRY, 41
P.: A man who asks you a lot of expensive ques-
tions   PSYCHIATRY, 8
the century of the p.'s couch   PSYCHIATRY, 37
The p. is the obstetrician of the mind PSYCHIATRY, 3
you need to retain a first-rate p. in today's world
                                           PSYCHIATRY, 7
psychiatrists P. classify a person as neurotic
                                           PSYCHIATRY, 43
The relation between p. and other kinds of lunatics
                                           PSYCHIATRY, 35
psychiatry P.'s chief contribution to philosophy
                                           PSYCHIATRY, 12
The new definition of p.   PSYCHIATRY, 2
psychic p. development of the individual
                           PSYCHIATRY, 20; PSYCHOLOGY, 6
the p. of human relationship between the sexes
                                           SEX, 14
psychoanalysis Considered in its entirety, p. won't
do.   PSYCHIATRY, 38
Freud is the father of p.   PSYCHIATRY, 27
plastic surgery . . . combines . . . p., massage, and a
trip to the beauty salon   PLASTIC SURGERY, 2

P. cannot be considered a method of education
                                           PSYCHIATRY, 31
P. is a permanent fad   PSYCHIATRY, 17
P. is confession   PSYCHIATRY, 13
P. is spending 40 dollars an hour   PSYCHIATRY, 15
P. is the disease it purports to cure PSYCHIATRY, 34
psychoanalyst The man who once cursed his fate . . .
pays his p.   PSYCHIATRY, 25
psychoanalysts I doubt whether p. would now maintain   PSYCHIATRY, 18
P. are not occupied with the minds of their patients
                                           PSYCHIATRY, 9
psychologist An animal p. is a man who pulls habits
out of rats.   PSYCHOLOGY, 1
psychology Idleness is the parent of all p.
                                           PSYCHOLOGY, 11
Popular p. is a mass of cant   PSYCHOLOGY, 4
P. is as unnecessary as directions for using poison
                                           PSYCHOLOGY, 8
P. . . . long past, . . . short history. PSYCHOLOGY, 5
p. should have destroyed . . . human nature
                                           PSYCHOLOGY, 2
P. which explains everything   PSYCHOLOGY, 10
the dull craft of experimental p.   PSYCHOLOGY, 14
The object of p. is to give us a totally different idea
                                           PSYCHOLOGY, 17
the popularity and persuasiveness of p.
                                           PSYCHOLOGY, 13
There is no p.   PSYCHOLOGY, 15
The separation of p. from the premises of biology
                                           PSYCHOLOGY, 7
psycho-pathologist the p. the unspeakable
                                           PSYCHIATRY, 36
psychotherapist time for the clergyman and the p. to
join forces   PSYCHIATRY, 30
psychotic A p. is the man who lives in it.
                                           PSYCHIATRY, 46
Psychiatrists classify a person as . . . p. PSYCHIATRY, 43
p. means he's even worse than my brother-in-law
                                           NEUROSIS, 9
The p. person knows that two and two make five
                                           NEUROSIS, 1
If a patient is poor he is committed . . . as p.
                                           PSYCHIATRY, 29
pulse The fingers should be kept on the p.
                                           DIAGNOSIS, 2
There are worse occupations in the world than feeling a woman's p.   DOCTORS, 94
There should be no doubt . . . as to . . . the meaning
of complexion and p.   DIAGNOSIS, 12
purse restore a man to his health, his p. lies open to
thee.   HEALTH, 3
Sickness soaks the p.   MEDICAL FEES, 17

quack By q. I mean imposter   QUACKS, 5
quackery Q. gives birth to nothing QUACKS, 1
quacks But modern q. have lost the art   MEDICAL
                                                 FEES, 8
Q. are the greatest liars in the world QUACKS, 2
Q. in medicine, . . . know this, and act upon that
knowledge.   QUACKS, 4
The practice of physic is jostled by q. on the one
side   QUACKS, 3
quadrangle the q. of health   HEALTHY LIVING, 21
quaffing Long q. maketh a short lyfe   DRINKING, 26
quiet Doctor Diet, Doctor Q. and Doctor Merryman
                                           DOCTORS, 96

People should be very free with s.   SEX, 13
poor honest s., like dying, should be a private matter.   SEX, 8
promiscuous s. in and out of season.   SEX, 17
S. is one of the nine reasons for reincarnation
                                                  SEX, 24
s. plays a more important part in the life of woman
                                                WOMEN, 25
sexes the psychic of human relationship between the
s.   SEX, 14
sexual Civilized people cannot fully satisfy their s. instinct without love   SEX, 31
He who immerses himself in s. intercourse will be
assailed by premature ageing   SEX, 22
The discussion of the s. problem   SEX, 14
sexuality S. is the lyricism of the masses.   SEX, 3
shadows The s. that I feared so long   BLINDNESS, 2
sick A person seldom falls s.   HUMAN NATURE, 1
Are you s., or are you sullen   HOLISTIC MEDICINE, 6
a s., its prison   BODY, 1
Be not slow to visit the s.   ILLNESS, 2
Every man who feels well is a s. man   ILLNESS, 26
He that eats till he is s.   HEALTHY EATING, 8
I deny the lawfulness of telling a lie to a s. man
                                    DOCTORS AND PATIENTS, 5
If you are physically s.   MENTAL ILLNESS, 19
if you don't object if I'm s.   SMOKING, 3
In the old-fashioned days when a man got s.
                                              TREATMENT, 13
I only take money from s. people.   HYPOCHONDRIA, 2
It is dainty to be s.   ILLNESS, 7
what he or his s. child needs is not medicine
                                         HEALTHY LIVING, 27
I will use treatment to help the s.   MEDICAL ETHICS, 5
medicines when well used restore health to the s.
                                             TREATMENT, 14
she cheats the s. and the dying with illusions
                                                NATURE, 10
S. minds must be healed as well as s. bodies
                                      HOLISTIC MEDICINE, 8
so many poor s. people in the streets full of sores
                                             EPIDEMICS, 5
The multitude of the s.   ILLNESS, 8
There is no curing a s. man   CURES, 1
The s. are the greatest danger for the healthy
                                             ILLNESS, 19
the s. man hands you gold in return   MEDICAL FEES, 3
The s. man is a parasite of society   INVALIDS, 2
The s. man is the garden of the physicians   DOCTORS
                                        AND PATIENTS, 12
a Hospital . . . should do the s. no harm.
                                            HOSPITALS, 10
'Tis healthy to be s. sometimes   HEALTH, 21
To be s. is to enjoy monarchal prerogatives.
                                              ILLNESS, 12
To heal the s.   MEDICAL STUDENTS, 10
To prevent disease, to relieve suffering and to heal
the s.   DOCTORS, 62
Treat the man who is s.   TREATMENT, 12
we think we're s.   MIND AND BODY, 9
you usually find that you are s.   MIND AND BODY, 2
sickness As s. is the greatest misery   ILLNESS, 5
Bathe early every day and s. will avoid you.
                                              HYGIENE, 4
He learns to depend on the physician in s. and in
health   HEALTH CARE, 1
How s. enlarges the dimensions of a man's self
                                             ILLNESS, 13
In s., respect health principally   HEALTH, 2

s. enlarges the dimensions of a man's self
                                         HYPOCHONDRIA, 10
S. is felt   ILLNESS, 23
S. is single trouble for the sufferer   NURSING, 3
S. soaks the purse.   MEDICAL FEES, 17
S. tells us what we are   ILLNESS, 24
Study s. while you are well   MEDICINE, 18
the greatest misery of s. is *solitude*   ILLNESS, 5
The problem of economic loss due to s.   HEALTH
                                                CARE, 4
The superior doctor prevents s.   DOCTORS, 19
To avoid s., eat less   HEALTHY LIVING, 8
weary thing is s.   ILLNESS, 9
sight should I not bear gently the deprivation of s.
                                            BLINDNESS, 5
s. is the most perfect and most delightful of all our
senses   SIGHT, 1
sightless When I was s. I cared for nothing
                                            BLINDNESS, 1
sign the s. 'Members Only'   SEX, 25
silver S. and gold have I none   CURES, 4
simpletons The world is so full of s. and madmen
                                       MENTAL ILLNESS, 25
sin A branch of the s. of drunkenness   DRINKING, 22
disease is the result of s.   TREATMENT, 18
the s. is on the head of all three   ABORTION, 6
sink The s. is the great symbol of the bloodiness of
family life   FAMILY, 3; NEUROSIS, 10
sister Too often a s. puts all her patients back to bed
                                              NURSING, 1
sit men s. and hear each other groan   HUMAN
                                            CONDITION, 3
sixty Men come of age at s.   AGE, 13
sixty-five I have been drinking it for s. years and I
am not dead   HEALTHY LIVING, 32
skeptics Half-informed physicians are generally s.
                                             DOCTORS, 24
skill Wonderful is the s. of a physician   MEDICAL
                                               FEES, 20
skin S. is like wax paper   SKIN, 2
Woollen clothing keeps the s. healthy   SKIN, 3
sleave ravell'd s. of care   SLEEP, 16
sleep A good laugh and a long s. are the best cures
                                               CURES, 18
haven't been to s. for over a year   SLEEP, 21
S. and watchfulness . . . when immoderate, constitute disease   SLEEP, 7
S. is better than medicine   SLEEP, 14
S. is gross   SLEEP, 6
S. is that golden chaine that ties health and our
bodies together   SLEEP, 3
s. is the condition to produce it.   SLEEP, 4
S. is when all the unsorted stuff comes flying out
                                               SLEEP, 5
s.! it is a gentle thing   SLEEP, 2
S. that knits up the ravell'd sleeve   SLEEP, 16
S.'s the only medicine that gives ease   SLEEP, 17
That sweet, deep s., so close to tranquil death
                                               SLEEP, 20
The amount of s. required by the average person
                                               SLEEP, 1
The beginning of health is s.   SLEEP, 8
the Lord God caused a deep s. to fall upon Adam
                                          ANAESTHESIA, 1
sleeping All this fuss about s. together   SEX, 35
slepe S. is the nourishment   CHILD CARE, 14
smart you had better be too s. to get ill   MEDICAL
                                                FEES, 1

smoke A woman is only a woman, but a good cigar
is a s. SMOKING, 17
Don't screw around, and don't s. HEALTHY LIVING, 10
I have seen many a man turn his gold into s.
SMOKING, 6
I s. almost constantly LONGEVITY, 8
resembling the horrible Stygian s. of the pit
SMOKING, 12
S., my friend SMOKING, 21
when I don't s. I scarcely feel as if I'm living
SMOKING, 11
smokers S., male and female, inject and excuse idle-
ness SMOKING, 5
smoking he had read of the effects of s. SMOKING, 22
resolve to give up s., drinking and loving
ABSTINENCE, 1
s. cigars and . . . drinking of alcohol before, after,
and . . . during ABSTINENCE, 3
S. . . . is a shocking thing SMOKING, 13
s. is one of the leading causes of statistics
SMOKING, 18
the beginning of the s. era. SMOKING, 2
The second week, he cut out s. HYPOCHONDRIA, 1
To cease s. is the easiest thing I ever did
SMOKING, 26
What a blessing this s. is SMOKING, 9
why he doesn't stop s. SMOKING, 23
snore s. and you sleep alone SNORING, 1
snorer can't hear himself s. SNORING, 2
soap Man does not live by s. alone HYGIENE, 3
S. and water and common sense ANTISEPTICS, 2
social We see the physician as scientist, educator and
s. worker DOCTORS, 92
society an age in which human s. dared to think of
the whole human race HEALTHY LIVING, 30
The sick man is a parasite of s. INVALIDS, 2
sociology The technology of medicine has outrun its
s. SCIENCE, 4
Sodom the men of S. were wicked HOMOSEXUALITY, 1
solicitude he will not frustrate himself further with
ineffective s. INCURABLE DISEASE, 1
solitary Life is for each man a s. cell LIFE, 18
Man is not a s. animal MANKIND, 27
solitude the greatest misery of sickness is s. ILLNESS, 5
soothe put you to sleep, wake you up, stimulate and
s. you all in one DRUGS, 19
sores Though physician . . . himself full of s.
DOCTORS, 47
sorrow in s. thou shalt bring forth children BIRTH, 3
soul A healthy body is the guest-chamber of the s.
BODY, 1
Body and s. cannot be separated for purposes of
treatment HOLISTIC MEDICINE, 4
Disease is . . . the result of conflict between s. and
mind DISEASE, 2
it must be inspired with s. MEDICINE, 24
My s. is full of whispered song BLINDNESS, 2
Nowhere can man find a quieter . . . retreat than in
his own s. MEDITATION, 5
The body is truly the garment of the s. BODY, 3
The human body is the best picture of the human s.
BODY, 15
the physicians separate the s. from the body HOLISTIC
MEDICINE, 9
The s. hath not her generous aspirings SMOKING, 19
The s. is subject to health and disease MIND AND
BODY, 5
when the s. is oppressed so is the body HOLISTIC
MEDICINE, 7

souls So long as our s. and personalities are in har-
mony DISEASE, 2
their s. dwell in the house of tomorrow CHILD CARE, 9
You may house their bodies but not their s. CHILD
CARE, 9
specialist A general practitioner can no more become
a s. GENERAL PRACTITIONERS, 2
A medical chest s. is long-winded about the short-
winded CONSULTANTS, 5
called a nerve s. because it sounds better
PSYCHIATRY, 49
Choose your s. and you choose your disease
CONSULTANTS, 3
No man can be a pure s. CONSULTANTS, 14
S. – A man who knows more and more about less
and less CONSULTANTS, 11
The s. is a man who fears the other subjects.
CONSULTANTS, 7
specialists Given one well-trained physician . . . than
ten s. CONSULTANTS, 12
species Pain is the correlative of some s. of wrong
PAIN, 20
S. do not evolve toward perfection EVOLUTION, 21
Women exist . . . solely for the propagation of the s.
WOMEN, 24
spectacles Putting on the s. of science SCIENCE, 3
speculation Medicine is a strange mixture of s. and
action. MEDICINE, 28
speed S. in operating should be the achievement
SURGEONS, 20
spermatozoa million million s., All of them alive
CONCEPTION, 2
spider do not be like the s., man HYPOCHONDRIA, 9
spirit There's nought . . . so much the s. calms
DRINKING, 12
those perish who lose their s. and energy HOLISTIC
MEDICINE, 4
spirits it quickly destroys both health and s.
MASTURBATION, 2
spiritual a symptom of some ailment in the s. part.
DISEASE, 7
spiritualist If the dead talk to you, you are a s.
SCHIZOPHRENIA, 3
spontaneous Worrying is the most natural and s. of
. . . functions WORRY, 3
spook medicine still falls somewhere between trout
casting and s. writing. MEDICINE, 22
sport kill us for their s. DEATH, 66
sports the childish nature will require s. CHILD
CARE, 15
spring In the s. . . . . your lovely Chloë YOUTH, 7
stages The four s. of man AGE, 9
stamp the indelible s. of his lowly origin EVOLUTION, 6
statistics Medical s. are like a bikini STATISTICS, 1
smoking is one of the leading causes of s.
SMOKING, 18
There are two kinds of s. STATISTICS, 2
steal all of his patients being willing to s. MEDICAL
FEES, 12
stench he begins as dirt and departs as s. MANKIND, 32
sterile human females become s. in the forties
FERTILITY, 4
still A s. small voice SUICIDE, 29
stimulant a good, cheap s. would be almost as popular DRUGS, 13
stimulate put you to sleep, wake you up, s. and
soothe you DRUGS, 19
stomach a little wine for thy s.'s sake DRINKING, 10
my s. must just digest in its waistcoat DRINKING, 40

The first possibility of rural cleanliness lies in *w. supply.* HYGIENE, 7
W., air, and cleanliness are the chief articles in my pharmacopoeia HEALTHY LIVING, 20
w. flowed like champagne ABSTINENCE, 5
w., honey, and labour REMEDIES, 20
wax Skin is like w. paper SKIN, 2
weak I inhabit a w., frail, decayed tenement ILLNESS, 1
The w., . . . always prevail over the strong EVOLUTION, 21
they are w. men NARCOTICS, 9
weakness private universe of physical w. and mental decay OLD AGE, 26
the strengths and w. of humanity so completely laid bare. DOCTORS, 57
wealth All health is better than w. HEALTH, 18
weariness The w., the fever, and the fret HUMAN CONDITION, 3
weed that tawney w. tobacco SMOKING, 14
week see what can be accomplished in a w. INCURABLE DISEASE, 3
well Every man who feels w. is a sick man ILLNESS, 26
fast till he is w. HEALTHY EATING, 8
Is getting w. ever an art CURES, 19
Living w. and beautifully and justly HEALTHY LIVING, 28
men who do not feel quite w. ILLNESS, 10
The fact that your patient gets w. DIAGNOSIS, 16
The skilful doctor treats those who are w. PREVENTIVE MEDICINE, 1
whim The strangest w. SUICIDE, 7
whisky A good gulp of hot w. at bedtime COUGHS AND COLDS, 7
whole A bodily disease, . . . w. and entire within itself DISEASE, 7
they are ignorant of the w. HOLISTIC MEDICINE, 9
They that be w. need not a physician ILLNESS, 3
wicked the men of Sodom were w. HOMOSEXUALITY, 1
wifehood w. and motherhood are but incidental relations WOMEN, 27
will he says 'I w.', he comes to his own as a philosopher MANKIND, 30
wine a little w. for thy stomach's sake DRINKING, 10
Drink w., and have the gout GOUT, 14
full of new w. DRINKING, 6
if you drink w. you have the gout GOUT, 16
look not thou upon the w. when it is red DRINKING, 9
that w. could derange its functions? DRINKING, 19
the w. is in, the wit is out DRINKING, 4
the red w. of Shiraz into urine? MANKIND, 6
w. is a mocker DRINKING, 8
W. is the most healthful DRINKING, 30
wisdom Self-reflection is the school of w. MEDITATION, 2
There is more w. in your body BODY, 11
W. not. KNOWLEDGE, 2
w. says: 'We must die,' LIFE AND DEATH, 9
wit wine is in, the w. is out DRINKING, 4
witchcraft Medical science is . . . imperfectly differentiated from . . . w. MEDICINE, 52
witches In the past, men created w. MENTAL ILLNESS, 51
woe Life protracted is protracted w. LONGEVITY, 5
w. unto them that . . . follow strong drink DRINKING, 7
woman An ailing w. lives forever WOMEN, 26
a w. is a w. SEX, 2

A w. is only a w., but a good cigar is a smoke SMOKING, 17
A w. should be an illusion. WOMEN, 10
God created w. WOMEN, 20
he has studied anatomy and dissected at least one w. DISSECTION, 2
It is almost a pity that a w. has a womb WOMEN, 2
Medicine is like a w. who changes with the fashions FADS, 1
One is not born a w. WOMEN, 4
sex plays a more important part in the life of w. WOMEN, 25
Six men give a doctor less to do than one w. WOMEN, 22
the anxiety of being a w. WOMEN, 5
The surgical cycle in w. WOMEN, 21
The years that a w. subtracts AGE, 3
To a physician, each man, each w. MEDICINE, 15
What does a w. want? WOMEN, 11
What is w. WOMEN, 8
When a w. becomes a scholar WOMEN, 18
w. is an animal that micturates once a day WOMEN, 16
W. is unrivaled as a wet nurse. WOMEN, 28
W. was God's *second* mistake. WOMEN, 20
womanhood The tobacco business is a conspiracy against w. and manhood SMOKING, 16
W. is the great fact in her life WOMEN, 27
womb How does a child live in the w. BODY, 5
It is almost a pity that a woman has a w. WOMEN, 2
mother's w. Untimely ripp'd BIRTH, 18
wombs when they feel the life of a child in their w. ABORTION, 1
women in w. nine out of ten abdominal swellings are the pregnant uterus PREGNANCY, 3
I think of w., it is their hair WOMEN, 19
Surgeons and anatomists see no beautiful w. ANATOMY, 5
the man who does not know sick w. does not know w. WOMEN, 17
we cannot instruct w. as we do men in the science of medicine WOMEN, 6
W. are equal because . . . not different WOMEN, 13
W. are most fascinating between the ages of thirty-five and forty WOMEN, 9
W. are so opinionated. WOMEN, 23
W. exist . . . solely for the propagation of the species WOMEN, 24
w., never. WOMEN, 3
word I would never use a long w. JARGON, 13
the addition of a new w. to the English vocabulary. JARGON, 11
words A man of true science . . . uses but few hard w. JARGON, 18
Whenever ideas fail, men invent w. JARGON, 7
work an environment equally fit for birth, growth w., healing, and dying HEALTHY LIVING, 14
W. and love – these are the basics NEUROSIS, 14
W. is the grand cure of all the maladies WORK, 1
world he must view the man in his w. HOLISTIC MEDICINE, 2
Into the dangerous w. I leapt BIRTH, 6
the credit goes to the man who convinces the w. RESEARCH, 10
The madman thinks the rest of the w. crazy. MENTAL ILLNESS, 47
The W. would be a safer place SCIENCE, 8
worry Eat everything, drink everything and don't w. about anything DRINKING, 43

NAME INDEX